PRAISE FOR WHY DIETS ARE FAILING US!

❝Peter Greenlaw's revolutionary nutritional technology helped me lose 15 pounds quickly. It has also dramatically improved my athletic performance. I am a believer!❞

Dr. William Andrews
THE WORLD'S LEADING PIONEER IN ANTI-AGING

❝Peter Greenlaw has lectured at over 1,000 forums in many Countries, educating people on **Toxicity**, **Obesity**, and **Living a healthy and Longer Life**.

The authors have included Important environmental information on toxic exposure, and the link between toxicity and obesity. This book is the most comprehensive explanation of todays challenges and the answers to better health.

Peter and Drew Greenlaw, and Dr Dennis Harper have over 28 years of combined experience in medically proven techniques and applied science providing answers to rid your body of dangerous and hazardous toxins which allow you to loose the weight you desire safely while improving your health. They have worked with thousands of patients using the latest cleansing techniques combined in a step by step system.

There is no other book that gives step by step instructions and discloses the hidden secrets you have been looking for. I urge you to read this book and learn how easy it is to have more energy, better health, more endurance, achieve your weight goal, and look and feel younger than you ever dreamed possible.❞

John W Anderson
NUTRACEUTICAL RESEARCH SCIENTIST

WHY **DIETS** ARE **FAILING** US!

Why Diets Are Failing Us!

Printed in the United States of America

First Printing, 2012

ISBN 978-0-9882771-1-3

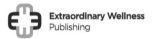 **Extraordinary Wellness** Publishing

Extraordinary Wellness Publishing
P.O. Box 123
Denver, CO 80205

www.HowDietsAreFailingUs.com

WHY DIETS ARE FAILING US!

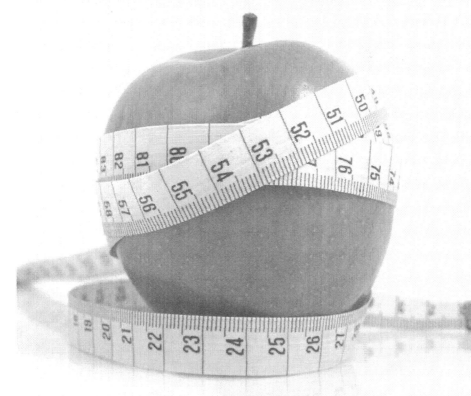

THE NEW WAY TO BE HEALTHY
AND LOSE WEIGHT

BY
PETER GREENLAW, DR. DENNIS HARPER, DREW GREENLAW

Acknowledgment

I want to give my sincere thanks to the following people who without their help this book would never have been completed:

John Anderson, the world's greatest nutritional formulator, who taught me so much about the remarkable nutritional technology he invented.

Jim and Kathy Coover, without whose vision, none of this would have been possible.

Tony and Randy Escobar, my first mentors, who took me by the hand and encouraged me to continue researching.

David Despain, M.Sc., who helped me get the science right.

My co-authors: Dr. Dennis Harper, for his incredible medical knowledge and guidance, and my son Drew, who was so instrumental in completing this book.

Jennifer Coulter, my editor who without her help I am not sure I ever would have finished.

And to my other son colin whose personal challenges were a huge motivator in writing this book in the first place.

And most importantly my wife sarah without her love and support I would never be where I am today.

    –Peter Greenlaw
     August 2012

Contents

Foreword

Peter Greenlaw has a passion for the best nutrition because he has learned the hard way when, despite his athletic background, and his continuing attention to good nutrition, his health gave out.

Not surprising, he learned that keeping the body healthy as we age is not as simple as it sounds in the media. Thankfully he found the right information, because that is what life is about—the right information.

Everything we know we learned from someone else. Were you born into a different culture, you would speak a different language, wear different clothes, follow different customs, and worship different gods. Yet they would be as true, and natural, and right to you as the beliefs you now hold most dear.

You have power to spare, given to you by creation as a gift right inside your genes, to develop a magnificent long and healthy life. All it takes is learning the right information to express that power. I urge you to study this book in order to achieve it.

–Michael Colgan, Ph.D., April 2012
Biochemist and Physiologist Nutritionist

Preface

Most of us face a variety of challenges related to weight management, health and wellness. My own personal story is one of a dramatic turnaround in my own health almost 10 years ago. The reason I am writing this book is to share my life-changing journey and a revolutionary approach to weight management and wellness with you. It is the reason I believe that I am still on this amazing planet that we all share.

Although the title of the book, "Why Diets Are Failing Us," suggests that I am only focusing on weight management, you'll find much more than that within these pages.

Since my own life-altering experience, I have helped tens of thousands of people regain their most important asset: their health. I even helped many of them win—for the first time—a victory in the battle against obesity once and for all. I did it by sharing this life-changing and incredible breakthrough in nutritional science in more than 1,000 lectures to audiences all around the world. Now, I want to share it with you through this book. Please know that I am not suggesting there is a "one size fits all" program. Rather, there are some excellent options to consider and adapt to your own body, lifestyle and personality.

There are more diet and exercise programs in the United States than ever before. Everywhere you look there are ads, commercials and articles about losing weight. According to the Center for Disease Control and Prevention (CDC), more than two thirds of Americans over age 20 are overweight, while one third are obese. It begs the question: Are diets working? If not, then what does? As a species we are not designed to be overweight, tired or unhealthy.

This book focuses on three key principles: to live healthier, to live longer and to maximize human potential. Even if you are already in great shape, I can promise you that it's in your genes to improve your overall health even further. If you have been doing the best you can based on the information available about health, nutrition and diets, but you can't seem to make progress, consider that you may be missing an important component.

One of the biggest factors that diets and exercise don't work as well as they have in the past is because our world has become more polluted. For example, even if you consume adequate servings of fruits and vegetables on a daily basis, you are still ingesting significant amounts of various chemicals. Every day we are exposed to chemicals from industrial waste, vehicle exhaust, food packaging, chemically treated water, pesticides, household cleaners, plastics and more.

There is now overwhelming evidence from the National Human Adipose Tissue Survey (EPA, 1990) that demonstrates that toxins are being stored in our fat tissue at a rapid rate. Sadly, they can also be passed on to the next generation as demonstrated by studies on umbilical cords of newborns. The placenta acts as an osmotic pump to deliver nutrients to the fetus from the mother. Now, we find this osmotic pump is carrying toxins and impurities as well.

In a study of umbilical cord blood of newborn babies, up to 287 toxic chemicals were noted in the umbilical cord blood (Houlihan, Kropp, Wiles, Gray, & Campbell, 2005). If babies have this amount of toxic chemicals in their bodies at birth, imagine how many we must have in our adipose fat tissue that is accumulating each and every day as adults.

Many of these chemicals are included under the umbrella term chronic "obesogens." These obesogens disrupt normal metabolism and contribute to obesity (Grun & Blumberg, 2006).

The American Society of Endocrinologists suggests that obesogens (Grun & Blumberg, 2006) are a major contributing factor in the dramatic increase of failing health and the epidemic of obesity. The term "obesogen" was first used by Felix Grun and Bruce Blumberg of the University of California, Irvine, to explain how toxins change the way our metabolisms work and contribute to obesity and poor health. Conventional diets simply do not offer any protection against obesogens, and are the reason diets are failing us. Diets simply fail in this polluted world. Healthy eating and exercising are no longer enough to avoid the toxins that are entering our bodies with the foods we eat, the air we breathe and the water we drink.

What can we do to reduce our toxic load and therefore our waistlines? The first step is to commit to becoming responsible for our own health and safety. We have one body to last us a lifetime; there are no spares.

I want to share a centuries-old revolutionary approach that changed my life and many others lives. This approach gave me real hope to win the battle against obesity. It is possible to release excess fat and keep it off while experiencing tremendous improvements in energy and overall feelings about life. I know because I've been there.

In this book I'll share with you the story of my health challenges and how I overcame them. I'll also give you information that will show you how and why conventional diets don't work in the long term. The scientific information is offered to you so you can understand the mechanisms in the body that create ill health and obesity. I will also offer you several paths toward achieving a healthier lifestyle that include cleansing and enjoying a nutrient-rich daily program. The programs allows you to jump-start your system with an 11-day nutritional cleansing program[1], or a more gradual 30-day nutritional cleansing program—with results that can't compare to conventional diets. At the end of the book, I will tell you about a free coaching system with qualified coaches and a program to ensure you have multiple solutions to fit your individual goals.

Whether you have 10 or 100 pounds to lose, are an athlete wanting to greatly increase the effectiveness of your workouts, or want more energy and less stress in your daily life, there is a program to fit your individual needs. This program's motto is "progress, not perfection." The path toward a healthy lifestyle must be taken one step at a time, and even the smallest steps and lifestyle changes can lead to vast improvements in your well-being.

---

1 This is the Isagenix 9-Day Cleanse and 2-Day Pre-Cleanse.

I invite you to consider the information presented in this book and make your own decisions. If you choose to take on the challenges and techniques in this book, and do what is recommended, you will increase the odds of living healthier longer while maximizing your human potential. This book will help you decide if this program is right for you, because only you can make the changes needed to live a healthier and more fulfilling life.

Wishing you vibrant health!

Peter Greenlaw
August 2012

Chapter 1 ———————
My Story

Today, I am strong, healthy and energetic—but I wasn't always like this. I had severe medical challenges that rocked me to my core and severely limited me.

My story starts with what I thought was a routine analysis of my yearly physical lab results more than nine years ago. It turned out that there was nothing routine about what my doctor was sharing with me. I thought, "This cannot be possible." The previous year everything was normal. There had to be a mistake.

I was about to learn there was no mistake. I felt myself literally shaking inside as my doctor went over the lab reports. Fear, anxiety and so many other emotions flooded me at that moment. My whole world was turned into an unbelievable nightmare in just five minutes in my doctor's office. What was I going to do?

My doctor's stern and scary advice was to lose 40 pounds, go on a vigorous exercise and diet program, and use Lipitor. If not, he warned, I would not see my kids graduate from high school. That was all the motivation I would ever need. At the time I was only 57 years old.

In my youth, I had worked out as a world class athlete as a member of the University of Colorado Ski Team. So, when my doctor said diet and exercise were the answer, I figured I could beat this with diet, exercise, his help and prescription drugs. Despite having been diligent in following a very intense workout schedule and diet regimen, I was disappointed that I lost only eight pounds after two months of suffering.

At that point, I was introduced to a nutritional system that changed my life. I will be forever grateful to the man who invented it. The very first thing I thought as I looked at my scale was that somehow it had broken in four days. I was still skeptical but continued on.

From there, I lost 20 pounds. To my astonishment I went from a 42-inch waist to a 34-inch waist—a size I have maintained for the past nine years. In all, I lost more than 30 pounds and have kept them off ever since. More importantly, I continue to be free of the need for prescription drugs—a major triumph.

At the time, I was completely amazed, but now I do not consider my story that unusual. A clinical study based on the nutritional program I used reveals that the average weight loss for men and women is seven pounds in just 11 days. This is a remarkable feat if you have suffered through any diet and or exercise program, only to lose a pound a week.

Perhaps most amazingly, for the past nine years I have also been free of the need for prescription drugs. My story is like so many others that I have heard and witnessed over the past decade, I just had to share my findings.

My transformation motivated me to find out why this particular program worked and why every other diet I had tried failed me every time I tried them. It is based on real science developed over the course of more than 25 years and it is finally available to all of us at a critical time in the history of mankind.

I believe that if we do not embark on a revolutionary new approach to solve our obesity problem, there will not be enough doctors, drugs and hospitals to take care of the number of people suffering the long-term negative health effects that obesity brings.

Our planet is changing at a rapid pace. The race to become faster, stronger and smarter continues to challenge humans in every way. The advancements in technology during the past 20 years have been nothing short of remarkable. these advancements have caused a paradox: they've caused our overall health to decline. Some people have recognized this and formed groups like Slow Food, which is a nonprofit association formed to counter the rise of fast food and fast life, the disappearance of local food traditions and people's dwindling interest in the food they eat.

New information is discovered and revealed daily about the dangers of processed foods and sugar. So-called food is no longer perceived as a "quick fix" to accommodate a fast-paced lifestyle, but now "a given" on the expressway to poor health. Yet millions of people still succumb to the lure of this damaging food.

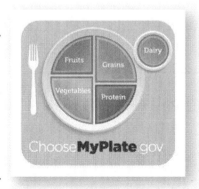

Also, there have been more than 20 scientific studies conducted over the past 30 years that show the formerly used USDA Food Pyramid and many of the dietary guidelines we have held as scientific fact are utterly false (in 2011 the Food Pyramid was changed to Choose My Plate). In fact, these supposed truths handed down from the government are actually damaging our health and making us fat and sick. Though significant medical and technological advancements have been made in recent years, the way people view their diet and nutrition has not kept pace with science. Instead, we rely on outdated knowledge and techniques that do not result in achieving optimum health.

Over the last century, milestone discoveries were made about the effects of vitamins and minerals on the body. For instance, revolutionary work by Nobel Prize-winning chemist Dr. Linus Pauling and his use of vitamin C opened the floodgates to understanding the beneficial effects of nutrients on the human body. Since then, products, supplements and diets have come and gone, yet we still know that vitamin and minerals have positive effects on the body's overall health.

Today, there are hosts of nutritional products available: CoQ10, vitamin A, B vitamins, and vitamin C and any number of individual nutrients. Many of these nutrients have positive effects on very specific locations in the body or facilitate specific processes such as circulation and cell division.

There are also many health techniques available. Cleanses eliminate parasites or aim to improve organ-specific functions—such as those in the liver, colon and gall bladder. I call these conventional nutrient solutions and cleansing processes "single-point-of-reference solutions."

What do I mean by single-point-of-reference solutions? Most nutrient formulations are created to deal with a specific need or concern in the body. The system for these solutions has not drastically advanced from those derived from Linus Pauling's original discovery of the effects of vitamin C on the body.

Considering this lack of progress, we need to get back to a simple fact: the body is an immensely complex system that needs to be treated as a whole. By focusing on an individual aspect or a singular ailment in the body, we are not discovering the real causes of our health issues.

Medicine is now dominated by hyper-focused specialists such as cardiologists, gastroenterologists, neurologists, dermatologists and many specialist surgeons who perform brain surgery, back surgery, heart surgery and even plastic surgery. Each of these specialists may prescribe different drugs or combinations of drugs to deal with all of these various systems within the body. For example, a diabetic who is prescribed insulin by an endocrinologist may see a cardiologist for drugs to combat high cholesterol and may be prescribed medicine by an internist to regulate high blood pressure caused by the disease.

These various individual drugs aimed at treating a single ailment in pinpointed locations throughout the body result in complex interactions and side effects. In reinforcing or treating one organ, each of these drugs, with their own cocktail of side effects, may be damaging others. It can also be damaging to take pharmaceutical drugs that mask symptoms. These can add toxins to the body without actually addressing the underlying cause. This isn't to say that some pharmaceutical drugs aren't important, but many people rely on them instead of looking at the root cause of their illnesses.

In essence, the body is a system that requires specialists to deal with all the sub-parts and specific organ systems that make up the entire human body. It is a very complicated chemical orchestration that requires special attention be given to each organ system in order for the body to function optimally as a whole.

Beyond needing different nutrients, vitamins and minerals for each of these organ systems, the body needs water for cooling and carrying out the complex neurological processes required for survival and cognitive functioning.

The human body, as a whole, is comprised of 60% water. The brain alone is 70% to 75% water and blood is 70% to 83% water. Yet even after consuming a wealth of vitamins, minerals and nutrients, most people are still deficient in the simplest and most abundant nutrient on earth: water. Water is just as vital a part of the whole as the other nutrients we need. Each one is a piece of a puzzle. All puzzle pieces rely on the next to complete the entire picture. We need each individual piece, but are we focusing too much on the individual pieces rather than the finished picture?

You cannot just live on one food source no matter how nutritious it is. The body requires a broad spectrum of nutrition from many food sources. For example, a diet of only apples would not supply your system with all that it needs to function for long-term wellness. Apples are nutritious, but they do not supply the body with the 51 nutrients the body requires to be nutritionally satisfied. Research says that if you lack just one of these 51 nutrients, it will never be satisfied, and you will never feel full no matter how much food you eat (Stitt, 1982). These nutrients are the bare minimum the body needs.

This is much like the state of nutritional science today, which has created these predominantly single-point-of-reference products to deal with specific areas of concern, and not the whole system. Although some have demonstrated notable results on their specific areas of focus, single-point-of-reference solutions—to fully treat a complex system—simply do not address the big picture. This is the dilemma that faces conventional nutritional science. Having focused on improving single-point solutions for decades we have severely overlooked the real issues.

Over the past five to six decades, failing health has continued to increase. Humans are in a downhill battle with our modern world and a new phenomenon has been introduced: "toxic burden." As technology, transportation and food production have improved over the years, these advancements have come at a certain cost all of human society and raise numerous questions and concerns. What are these chemicals doing to us? Why, in such an advanced society, is our general state of health in such decline?

Perhaps we need to be better educated about toxicity and nutrition. While there is a good deal of misinformation out there, many of us have adopted an "ignorance is bliss" attitude about our health. Though fast food is considered to be detrimental to our health and weight, people continue to eat it regularly, ignoring warning signs to the contrary. When we eat this way our bodies are forced to develop ways to protect itself from the toxicity and lack of nutrients in the food, as well as deal with an increasingly toxic world. In order to protect our vital organs, many of the body's security systems are based on the production of fat cells. Scientists have found that the body uses fat cells not only for storage, but also to provide extra protection from our modern world. As a result, we get fatter and fatter in an attempt to protect ourselves from our toxic world.

Most doctors, according to a recent survey, don't have the resources to deal with obesity. In a national survey of 290 primary care physicians conducted by Harris Interactive in 2009, 89% of primary care physicians believe it is their responsibility to help overweight or obese patients lose weight, but 72% of those surveyed also said that no one in their practice has been trained to deal with weight-related issues. These findings and others come from research commissioned and released by the Strategies to Overcome and Prevent (STOP) Obesity Alliance. The survey reveals that most physicians don't have many of the tools they need to help people succeed in losing weight (STOP Obesity Alliance Research Team, 2010).

Recently, a study by Duke University projected that 42% of Americans may end up obese by 2030, which is up from 36% in 2010. The increase in the obesity rate would mean 32 million more obese people within two decades (Finkelstein, 2012).

There is no argument that toxicity, obesity and stress lead to poor health and that poor health leads to accelerated aging and ultimately a shortened lifespan. There is a perpetual challenge in generating awareness and developing efficient solutions, despite the fact that obesity is known to contribute to more than 60 chronic diseases, including heart disease, Type 2 diabetes and many types of cancer.

There are answers out there; we just have to be willing to restructure our current belief systems about how and what to eat.

Achieving true health is all about nutritional density, nutritional calories and the balance of fats, carbohydrates and proteins. Cutting calories is no longer an efficient method when there is a foundational lack of nutrition. There are no "magic pills" that will melt the weight off without major side effects. To survive in this modern world, we all need to dedicate ourselves to learn from the past and move into the new frontier of nutritional science.

The bottom line is that we need to be educated on the real health issues we face in today's toxic world. Chemicals and pollutants are not going away; in fact, they are increasing every year. Obesity is becoming a pandemic for which populations are largely unprepared.

As you will see, there is a real long-term solution to this seemingly insurmountable problem that has plagued and baffled the medical community for many years.

Chapter 2 _____

Dieting: What Works, What Doesn't

"If fat is not an insidious creeping enemy, I do not know what is."
William Banting, Letter on Corpulence, Addressed to the Public (1869)

There are striking similarities between diets from hundreds of years ago and the diets we follow now. Very little has changed. But throughout the centuries the word "diet" has drastically morphed. Initially, the Greek word "diatia" suggested a sensible, moderate and dutiful way of living and originally had no specific reference to food, Later it came to be associated with foods that are customarily eaten. Though this definition is still used, "diet" is now indicative of an all-consuming practice and desire to lose weight—an $80 billion dollar industry that, according to the National Institute of Health, fails 98% of dieters. It summons images of fat-free rice cakes, diet sodas, restrictive meals, point systems, calorie counting and deprivation. But how did the dieting craze of today first begin?

Dieting goes back at least as far as the 3rd century BC, according to Louise Foxcroft, author of *Calories & Corsets: A History of Dieting Over 2000 Years*. She says that followers of the ancient Greek physician Hippocrates recommended a diet of light and emollient foods, slow running, hard work, wrestling, sea-water enemas, walking about naked and vomiting after lunch. The Greeks believed that being fat was morally and physically detrimental, the result of luxury and corruption, so food and living should be plain with nothing to unduly stir the passions or arouse the appetites. This was the first documented diet or "diatia" (Foxcroft, 2011).

It's rumored that in 1087, William the Conquerer had become too heavy to ride his horse and decided that he would stop eating solid foods and only partake in a "liquid diet" that consisted only of alcohol in an attempt to lose weight. If this tale is true, it's the first recorded example in which an individual changed his or her food habits to lose weight. Although it was never documented whether or not the diet worked, William later died from a horse accident. Since he was able to ride a horse, this has led historians to believe that the diet was somewhat successful (Gruber, 2002).

Since William's "liquid diet," thousands of diet theories have surfaced. Nearly 150 years ago, Englishman William Banting was advised by his doctor to begin journaling about his "diet" because he was not feeling healthy and noticed he had put on weight. What Banting did was not too different than what people do today; he cut sugars and starches from his meals. He was the first to record his progress in consuming a low-carbohydrate diet. He ate only protein (meat, poultry or fish), along with a combination of green vegetables and fruit. Banting lost 50 pounds in less than 12 months (Edwardes, 2003).

Remarkably, Banting's diet is almost identical to a famous diet that many people use today. This protocol remains one of the foundations of our conventional diet belief system. It follows the same pattern it did for Banting: average weight loss of around one pound per week.

Not long after the success of Banting's diet, merchants began marketing a variety of products to promote weight loss. It was not uncommon for these products to contain laxatives, purgatives, arsenic, strychnine, thyroid hormones, amphetamines and other unsafe ingredients. Although proven dangerous, people still believe they can successfully lose weight with these chemicals.

In 1917, the weight-loss industry began to focus on calories when Dr. Lulu Hunt Peters published *Diet and Health* (Peters, 1918). The success of her book was attributed to the concept of counting calories. It sold more than two million copies and became the first bestselling American diet book. Dr. Peters urged readers to view the calorie as a measurement and rather than judge meals by portion size. It was recommended that the amount of calories in any given food were counted and totaled each day. She concluded that to lose weight it was important to stay under 1,200 calories a day.

Since Dr. Peters successful book, there have been hundreds of popular diets that use calorie counting as the principle method of losing weight.

There is no doubt that counting calories has worked in the past. But modern-day calories have changed because the nutrition contained in a calorie has diminished. The calories that most of us consume are just not the same from a nutritional standpoint as calories consumed by people in the past. Though it can be argued that a high-calorie diet will cause weight gain and a low-calorie diet will lead to weight-loss, the body's health does not solely rely on this aspect of nutrition.

If the body is constantly supplied with calories that have no nutritional value, the body will want to eat more, causing weight gain, obesity and disease. Therefore, how does one fully nourish the body without overloading on calories? It is possible—and to understand the solution, it is necessary to explore the calorie and common beliefs surrounding it.

Calorie Counting: Fact vs. Fiction

Counting calories is the most common diet method among the estimated millions of Americans on diets today. One of the greatest misconceptions about weight loss is that reducing caloric intake will permanently reduce body weight. Unfortunately, the calorie has become the weight loss measuring stick for the consumption of food and nutrients. You know the drill—people who count calories are constantly counting, reducing, restricting and rearranging—all to achieve weight loss, better health and better well-being. But they are missing a critical component.

A calorie is a unit of energy. In the U.S., the popular use of the term calorie actually means the kilocalorie, sometimes called the kilogram calorie, or large Calorie (equal to 1,000 calories), in measuring the calorific, heating or metabolizing value of foods. Thus, the "calories" counted for dietary reasons are in fact kilocalories. This unit of measurement is the amount of heat required to raise the temperature of one kilogram of water one degree Celsius (Encyclopædia Britannica, 2012). The number of calories indicated for a given food expresses how much energy is supplied to the body in consuming it. Most health professionals and the general public associate calories with whatever they drink or eat. Calories cannot be directly equated to levels of nutrition.

Conventional diet companies, books and health education are firmly based upon the concept of restricting calories as a sure way to lose weight. The problem with this is calories cannot be measured in the body. They can only be measured in a laboratory setting. The human body cannot compute calories, it can only use what's available in order to function as efficiently as possible.

If all our calories came from foods like cookies, candies, ice cream and sodas, these calories would have seriously detrimental effects on the body. Too many calories from these simple sugars contribute to obesity and diabetes, along with numerous other diseases.

What would be the difference between our consumption of 1,200 calories per day from fruits and vegetables versus 1,200 calories per day from cookies and candy? Clearly, each diet consists of the same number of calories, but in the long run each would result in two very different outcomes for the body. Eating only sugars and carbohydrates would lead to poor health and looming obesity. It is the composition of the food that matters, not the calorie itself. So, instead of counting calories as a means of losing weight, we should measure the level of nutrition.

From his book, *The New American Diet*, Stephen Perrine agrees that the emphasis on the counting of calories is not the way to go. "We have plenty of things that look like "health food," low-fat cakes, low-carb cookies, juice boxes that claim their contents are made from "real fruit." But they're not actually food" (Perrine, 2010).

He says that these processed food products are packed with empty calories, not nutrients, and they do basically one thing: make you fat. For example, after you eat a big bowl of empty calories from a cardboard box, your body is still waiting for some actual nutrients. That's why we eat again when we should be full (Perrine, 2010).

Perrine agrees with the basic premise that it is not the concept of calories that is most important, but it's the nutrition in the calories we eat. We overeat because our bodies are starved for real nutrition. We eat more calories because our bodies are not satisfied with the amount of nutrition in the processed foods we eat. The focus should not be on the amount of calories consumed, but on the nutritional density of those foods.

In a perfect world, the food we eat would contain, at a minimum, the 51 nutrients we must have in order for the body to be nutritionally satisfied. Those nutrients would ideally be included in the fewest number of calories necessary to sustain us.

According to Paul Stitt, "Calorie intake is only one part of good nutrition. Dieters especially are prone to the misconception that calories are all they need to count, so they fill their meager caloric allowance with foods that are high in processed carbohydrates and almost devoid of other essential nutrients, foods which can only aggravate their hunger, yet never give their bodies what they really need. At the same time, the empty calories they eat rob their bodies of what nutrients they have stored" (Stitt, 1982).

Calories and nutrition are not one in the same. As nutrition becomes scarce in the calories that we consume, we need to concern ourselves with the absorption of the nutrients that exist in the foods we eat.

Only by achieving a balance in the nutrients absorbed into the body can the body's natural processes function normally and efficiently. Otherwise, we will continue to be overweight and undernourished.

According to some estimates there may be as many as 170 million Americans who are now overweight and nearly 34% of those are obese. The incidence of obesity in children under 14 doubles every six years and has reached epidemic proportions in the United States, and a pandemic worldwide (Ogden, C.; Carroll, M., 2010).

To combat this growing health crisis, it is critical that we make nutrition a part of the process. People need to refocus and look at balanced nutrition. Getting micronutrients such as vitamins and minerals into the body is the key to benefitting from what we eat.

Is Exercise and Diet the Only Answer?

With more than two-thirds of America overweight and more than 30% suffering from obesity it seem obvious that exercise and diets are failing us.

I have seen some estimates that say 80 to 90% of all diets are failing us. So many people are disappointed and keep waiting for the "miracle diet." But almost a century of research has shown that dieting—which usually involves calorie restriction—is not the way to lose weight and improve health. Repeatedly, studies have found that, while eating less causes short-term weight-loss, a majority of people on diet plans gain most of the weight back within one year, and the majority (90-95%) gain all of it back within three to five years (Mann, T. et al, 2007).

We are spending billions of dollars each year on diets that fail most of the time. The promise of weight loss is a great business. You can have a 90% failure rate and the customers keep coming! I was certainly part of this false hope that the ads portrayed. Eventually, I realized I was forcing myself to hope. Even though I had extreme motivation to lose weight, I had limited success. I am not sure I could have continued on the diet and exercise program prescribed by my doctor, scared as I was.

New diets keep appearing each year with fancy and creative names. Yet, after trying, the weight creeps back on and we are right back where we started. The Surgeon General states that more people will die this year from being overweight than those who smoke cigarettes and about 60 conditions are worsened by obesity, according to George Blackburn, Abraham Associate Professor of Nutrition at Harvard-affiliated Beth Israel Deaconess Medical Center.

Remember the disaster of approved "miracle" diet drugs that ended up severely injuring—and in some cases—killing those who took them? Some of these victims even took them under a doctor's supervision. Something is terribly wrong. Solution after solution does not seem to get us any closer to solving this obesity epidemic. It only seems to be getting worse.

What About Exercise?

In addition to diet, exercise is peddled as the missing link to successful weight loss. Although exercise supports overall health and wellness, I was shocked to learn that many experts say that it does not work as a lone strategy for losing weight. Though maintaining an active lifestyle has proven to help people live longer and healthier lives, exercise is not the sole solution and is only one of the keys to weight loss.

"Exercise does not help lose weight in most people but only helps to not gain any pounds. This is somewhat profound and makes you realize that if someone truly wants to lose weight, it is by improving the resting metabolic rate that you can hope to succeed. If toxins can (and they do) impair this process, we need to discover ways to improve that mechanism through detoxification and toxin avoidance" (Schauss, 2008).

As you know, I had a similar personal experience. After two months of killing myself in the gym with routines that most people would never attempt I had lost only eight pounds. There was no way I would have kept up that extreme exercise routine with such little to show for it.

If diet and exercise are not working the way we've been taught, what is the answer?

Chapter 3 ⸻

Toxins: The Good and the Bad

We are continually exposed to natural toxins and synthetic chemicals every day—in the food we eat, air we breathe, water we drink and items we touch. Learning more about these harmful impurities is critical for making decisions to protect our long-term health.

Although we normally think of toxins only as synthetic chemicals, natural toxins have always been part of the environment. Many natural toxins are produced by plants, bacteria and animals as defenses to keep predators at bay. This natural arms race has produced millions of different toxins, including venoms and poisons, as a means of protecting the life of an individual species. One example of a toxin is caffeine. Plants began producing caffeine as a way to disorient insects that try to eat the plant (Weinberg & Bealer, 2001). The creatures eating the caffeine were more likely to forget what they ate or avoid the plant all together due to the caffeine high. It could be argued that caffeine could produce the same results in humans. In fact, NASA labs have identified caffeine as the chemical most responsible for human error (Wilkinson, 1995).

Human exposure and reaction to these natural toxins depends largely on how food is prepared. Cooking food breaks down many plant and animal (toxic) defenses. Also, the process of fermentation, in which microorganisms predigest a food to make it more edible, also acts to disintegrate them. According to Sally Fallon, author of *Nourishing Traditions*, almost all traditional societies used fermented and cultured processes to enhance the enzyme content of some foods and break down enzyme inhibitors. For example, without fermentation and cooking, grains and legumes are not easily digested (Fallon, 2001). Heat and fermentation can also make food safe by neutralizing plant toxins and destroying detrimental bacteria.

Still, the introduction of new foods and food preparation techniques throughout history has generated toxins and chemicals. For example, when heat is used to cook meat the reaction can emit its own chemicals, such as char and nitrosamines. And, while heat may break down the toxic defenses present in the food being cooked, the chemicals produced can have a carcinogenic toxic effect on the body.

Toxins are even produced within the human body from simply living day to day. Toxins may, at times, be produced to battle foreign bacteria and viruses. These can cause harm as they work to protect the body. But after their job is done, they are ultimately detoxified through biochemical processes.

All of these toxins are usually eliminated by the body without much adverse effect, but in our modern environment pollution and food processing have increased the body's toxic burden considerably. Humans have added thousands of new chemicals that pollute the air and water, which can often end up concentrated in foods. Beyond this, food is also laden with chemicals in the form of pesticides, processing agents, hormones, antibiotics and other artificial ingredients.

According to Mark Hyman, M.D., in his book *The Ultra Mind Solution*, "The average person consumes one gallon of neurotoxic pesticides and herbicides each year by eating conventionally grown fruits and vegetables" (Hyman, 2009). By consuming any amount of conventionally grown fruits and vegetables, humans are at risk of harming their bodies. Since pesticides are neurotoxic and work by attacking insects' nervous systems, we may be similarly damaging our nerve processes by ingesting large quantities of toxic pesticides from our food and environment.

The continual flow of pollutants into water sources increases our risk of exposure to toxins as well. There are now hundreds of chemicals in municipal drinking water, including Prozac, Lipitor, and many other pharmaceutical and prescription drugs that may have adverse effects on the body and its functions. As the body is endlessly exposed, these toxins can overwhelm the body's natural detoxification defenses. A slow accumulation of toxicity in the body may eventually disturb its natural processes.

Even newborns have a toxic burden. In a 2005 study the Environmental Working Group (EWG) commissioned laboratory tests of 10 American Red Cross umbilical cord blood samples for the most extensive array of industrial chemicals, pesticides and other pollutants ever studied. The group found that the babies averaged 200 contaminants in their blood. The pollutants included mercury, fire retardants, pesticides and the Teflon® chemical PFOA. In total, the babies' blood had 287 chemicals, including 209 never before detected in cord blood (Environmental Working Group, 2005). Recent public tests conducted on adults in the industrialized world have shown that each person studied carries between 500 and 700 toxins in their bodies.

Furthermore, most of the foods available today are not designed to support our bodies nutritionally, and the ubiquitous oversized portions only add to our toxic burden. Overly busy schedules and strenuous lifestyles have made processed foods a convenient option, adding to our waistlines and increasing the body's level of toxicity.

The human body has had to adapt over generations to remove various toxic loads. The body is equipped with powerful detoxification and cleansing systems in the liver, stomach, intestines and kidneys as means of protecting itself. The liver is the primary detoxification organ, metabolizing thousands of different chemicals to which humans are exposed daily. Much of what is eaten must pass through the liver. As the liver breaks down nutrients, it also metabolizes toxic substances. In most cases, these toxins are cleared from the blood and eliminated in bile or urine, but at other times, they can be stored in fat.

The body stores these impurities in body tissues such as fat even as polluted elements continue to enter the body. The fat cells then enlarge because of additional fat. The toxins are solubilized with the fat. According to Mark Hyman, there are two types of toxins when it comes to storage in the body. There is water soluble or fat soluble. Water soluble toxins will be eliminated through urine and sweat. Fat soluble toxins will dissolve and recombine using fat (Hyman, 2009).

After extensive research in recent years, scientists have begun to realize that the long-term implications of toxins may result in drastic changes to the internal structure of the human body. The immune system is incapable of dealing with so many chemicals, and latest evidence shows that toxins disrupt metabolism. When the body does not metabolize effectively, this can lead to obesity. These chemicals are obesogens, or foreign chemical compounds that disrupt normal development and balance of fat metabolism.

The Endocrine Society, the largest organization of experts devoted to research on hormones and the clinical practice of endocrinology, reports that "the rise in the incidence in obesity matches the rise in the use and distribution of industrial chemicals that may be playing a role in a generation of obesity, suggesting Endocrine Disrupting Chemicals (EDCs) may be linked to this epidemic" (Perrine, 2010). Endocrine disrupting chemicals (EDCs) are a type of obesogen that is broadly defined as chemicals that can interfere with hormone action. These EDCs play havoc in our bodies in many ways. For example, it is now clear that other hormone receptor types and functions, including those involved in metabolism, obesity and brain signaling can be targets of EDCs (The Endocrine Society, 2009).

"Simply put, obesogens are chemicals that disrupt the function of our hormonal system, leading to weight gain and many of the diseases that curse the American populace. They enter our bodies from a variety of sources-from natural compounds found in soy products, from artificial hormones fed to our animals, from plastic pollutants in some food packaging, from chemicals added to processed foods, and from pesticides sprayed on our produce. They act in a variety of ways-mimicking human hormones such as estrogen, blocking the action of other hormones such as testosterone, and, in some cases, altering the functions of our genes and essentially programming us to gain weight" (Perrine, 2010).

Frederick vom Saal, Ph.D., curators' professor of biological science at the University of Missouri-Columbia has stated, "Obesogens are thought to act by hijacking the regulatory systems that control body weight" (vom Saal, F. et al, 2012). This presence of obesogens is the first reason that traditional dieting methods have become outdated. Never before have traditional, low-carbohydrate, low-calorie diets been forced to accommodate for this level of synthetic chemicals and the adverse effects they have on the body. The body's attempt to protect itself from the constant assault of synthetic toxins results in the production and storage of fat.

Scientists have also found that low levels of certain compounds, such as bisphenol A—the building block of hard, polycarbonate plastic, including that in baby bottles—have surprising effects on cells growing in lab dishes. Usually, cells become fibroblasts that make up the body's connective tissue. However, pre-fibroblasts have the potential to become adipocytes or fat cells. These studies show that bisphenol A, and some other industrial compounds pushed pre-fibroblasts to become fat cells and stimulated the proliferation of existing fat cells.

Scientist Jerry Heindel believes this has enormous implications. He says, "The fact that an environmental chemical has the potential to stimulate growth of pre-adipocytes has enormous implications. If this happened in living animals as it did in cells in lab dishes, the result would be an animal [with] the tendency to become obese." Heindel's studies also imply that a person's toxic burden can have consequences for three to four generations after the time of exposure.

"Researchers are reporting new data, both in animals and in humans, that indicate the effects of these chemicals can be seen not just in our bodies, but across three or four generations. So a pregnant woman affects her children, grandchildren, and great grandchildren" (Perrine, 2010).

The research on this generational battle is all without true regard for how the body is handling these high levels of poison. Major studies conducted by Mt. Sinai Medical School have shown that the body stores elements of pollution, acid and impurities in fat cells. In these studies, all participants tested positive for between 100 and 200 toxic chemicals in their blood and urine. None were free from some form of toxicity.

Considering all this information—the buildup of chemicals, pesticides and hormones in the body—it is heavily implied that a strong correlation exists between a person's toxic burden and the size of his or her waistline. These impurities may not only be helping the body to store fat, but they are changing the body's genetic structures to self-regulate.

Dr. Paula Baillie-Hamilton is a medical doctor and visiting fellow in occupational and environmental health at Stirling University in Scotland. She is also considered to be one of the world's leading authorities on toxic chemicals and their effects on our health. She believes that, "What appears to be happening is that our natural slimming system is being poisoned by the toxic chemicals we encounter in our everyday lives; and this damage is making it increasingly difficult for our bodies to control their weight. The end result is that we gain weight in the form of fat and not muscle, as chemicals tend to cause muscles to shrink and body fat to accumulate" (Baillie-Hamilton, 2005).

Michael Pollan, author of, *The Omnivore's Dilemma* and *In Defense of Food*, said it best when he pointed out that you are not only what you eat but, "You are what it eats too. If our beef is loaded with hormones that are designed to cause artificial weight gain, and we eat said beef… Wouldn't we be likely to gain unnatural amounts of weight too?" (Pollan, 2006). There must be a direct correlation between our weight gain and the synthetic hormones pumped into our food supplies. We may never turn into a "hot dog" but we may share the extra side of fat in that rib eye.

Due to the prevalence of pesticides, herbicides and antibiotics in food, very little of what humans eat can be fully broken down by the body. Instead these toxic elements are being stored as fat and ultimately contributing to the overall degeneration of the state of human health.

According to the FDA, there are now more than 100,000 chemicals in commercial use in this country. Only 560 of those have been tested for their health effects on humans. There is great concern among scientists and researchers about the combination of all of these chemicals forming new chemical compounds within the human body. What will the long-term effects be?

It's no longer speculation that today's toxic world is taking its toll on the human body. Winning the battle against a toxic present and future for the human race is much more complex than just eating healthy foods and counting empty calories. Conventional dieting and exercise methods are—at best—helping people to maintain their weight, but they are not providing the tools for permanent weight loss or vibrant health.

The first step is to become aware of the problem and avoid chemical-laden, processed, empty-calorie foods as much as possible. It's critical to avoid exposure to toxins when there is a choice to do so. It is also important to consume more water and avoid beverages that dehydrate your cells. But the solution requires more than just this basic understanding of the calorie, the effects of everyday toxins and how to eliminate them from the body. Armed with this knowledge, we can embark on a journey to find our best selves.

Chapter 4
High Quality Nutrients and Cleansing

In a perfect world, the body internally regulates every system at a high efficiency. If it needs to cleanse itself, it will. If it needs to burn off extra fat, it is designed to do so. The easiest way to burn fat is to stimulate the body's metabolism. To increase metabolism over time, the body needs highly nutritious sources of calories.

Because the body's hormonal and the natural processes have been confused by increased exposure to synthetic chemicals, artificial sweeteners and overall poor nutrition, we must change our eating habits to be healthy and maintain a reasonable body weight. Today's food largely lacks vitamins, minerals and enzymes, which are often destroyed in food preparation. Humans are consuming more calories in order to compensate for nutritionally barren food. Therefore, reducing our caloric intake can no longer be considered a reliable way to maintain health and achieve weight loss. Even food companies that put forth "fortified "or "enriched" products often substitute synthetic chemicals for naturally occurring nutrients that are no longer abundant in most foods.

Conventional dieting just does not make any sense anymore; yet there seems to be a new diet every week encouraging people to reduce calories to reduce their waistlines. However, reduced calories lead to a further reduction in nutrients, resulting in less protection against toxins and worsened health.

Scientists are now coming to the conclusion that most of our food supply is on its way to becoming almost nutritionally bankrupt. This includes a wide array of fruits and vegetables, in which some nutrients are almost nonexistent. This gets back to the whole idea that a calorie without nutrition is basically like eating air. This is why many people experience hunger after consuming huge quantities of nutritionally bankrupt, processed foods. And we wonder why we keep eating and eating. Well, it is because our body is looking for the nutrition that has vanished from our food.

In the book *Beating the Food Giants*, biochemist Paul A. Stitt provides evidence that supports the premise that calories should not be the standard by which we base our eating, health and longevity.

"The organ that controls our cravings for food is called the appestat. It is located at the base of the brain, possibly in the hypothalamus (an area of the pituitary gland). The appestat is constantly monitoring the blood for nutrient content. Only when 51 nutrients are present at their proper levels will the individual feel entirely full and satisfied. If anyone nutrient is missing, the individual feels hungry" (Stitt, 1982).

He continues with more scientific evidence about nutritional deficiencies effect on hunger.

In an extensive study on dietary relationships conducted by nutritionists Drs. R.A. Harte and B. Chow discovered that the absence of a single essential vitamin, mineral, amino acid or fatty acid can create a "shock wave" that hinders the metabolization of all other nutrients (Stitt, 1982).

Getting an improper nutrient balance can be almost as bad as getting no nutrients at all. It is important to remember that the body's hunger mechanism is affected by the presence of nutrients, not just calories. Although much more complex, the body works synergistically, like a car. A car can have a perfectly tuned engine, but without gasoline it won't run. Or a car can have a full tank of gasoline, but with a dead battery, it won't start. A car can have gasoline and a new battery, but if it has a flat tire it won't go very far. This is how the body works as a system. All the systems need to be functioning if we are to have optimal health, and to live healthier, longer.

Although there was a time for conventional methods of dieting, that time has passed. Too often, we continue to try these methods over and over, starving our bodies to lose a little weight—only to gain it back in a fourth of the time it took to lose it. This is such a discouraging cycle for anyone who has experienced it. Though this propensity for weight regain often makes us feel guilty, it's very likely that the dieting techniques themselves, and not our willpower, is to blame for the yo-yo weight loss and gain that is so common in this society. Those diets were based on a premise that may have worked 100 years ago, but they are not equipped to deal with the increased pollution, impurities and toxins (obesogens) of today's world.

The world is inundated with overly processed food, and because of fast-paced lifestyles and poor dietary choices, we often feel cornered into eating food products that are high in sugars and simple carbohydrates. The body consistently burns more 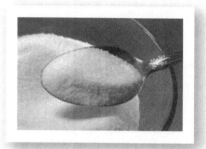 carbohydrates for energy than protein and fat, and an excess of sugar in the diet hinders the body's ability to burn fat. It is estimated that we consumed 131.9 pounds of sugar per person per year in 2010 (USDA, 2011). In the late 1800s, it was estimated that the average person consumed only 10 pounds of sugar in a year. These statistics don't account for the consumption of simple sugars found in fruits, but show comparatively that in just over a hundred years the average human's sugar consumption has multiplied by more than 13 times.

The way the body is designed to work is to burn fat, proteins and carbohydrates. During emergencies it turns to what is easily broken down, which is glucose and glycogen but it will also metabolize proteins as well during this time of emergency.

According to Dr. Dennis Harper, "The problem is the majority of us are in sugar burning mode most of the time because the foods that we eat are mostly high glycemic foods that contain lots of sugar" (Harper, 2012).

Though glucose is needed in certain doses so that the brain can function properly, the brain only requires four grams of pure glucose every three hours, which is slightly less than a teaspoon. Most people far surpass this on a daily basis. The problem is that if the body is forced to consistently burn excess amounts of sugar, an incredible toll will be taken on the body's efficiency and ability to function and develop.

"As soon as the body senses higher glucose levels the insulin levels will become much higher which can result in a hypoglycemic reaction that can increase adrenaline, a stress hormone called cortisol and another hormone called ghrelin" (Harper, 2012).

Higher glucose levels cause the body to counterattack by increasing insulin. The increased insulin lowers blood sugar (glucose), and we get hungry again. Low blood sugar causes us to crave carbs and other foods when our blood sugar gets low because the brain requires four grams of sugar every three hours to function properly.

When we get low on glucose we overcompensate and we crave foods that will temporarily make us feel better, but tend to be detrimental for our bodies in the long run. These high-calorie foods are frequently packed with simple sugars, which further complicates the process of traditional dieting by causing the body to enter a state of stress. When we're stressed our adrenal glands respond by increasing cortisol levels, the major stress hormone. Why is this detrimental to maintaining our weight and health?

According to Dr. Harper, "Higher levels of adrenaline are necessary if you are being chased by a bear or you are under a lot of stress. Cortisol is also increased under stress to increase the amount of fuel needed for the body. It is normally produced every night to help keep inflammation down and slowly goes down during the day. Higher levels associated with stress will reduce digestion, growth, reproduction and the immune system. Sugar consumption can cause higher levels of insulin, which may produce inflammation, hypo-glycemia, which then stresses the body and triggers an increase in adrenaline and cortisol, which is not desirable" (Harper, 2012).

Between an influx of the toxins and consumption of a surplus of sugar, the primary systems and functions of the body can slacken and become sluggish. As a result, we must search for new solutions to achieve long lasting health and weight loss that include being much more conscientious of the types and form of nutrients we ingest.

If conventional dieting methods and the old concept of "healthy eating" are no longer enough to maintain a healthy weight, then how should we eat? How can we be mindful and restrict caloric intake without suffering greater nutrient deficiency? How can fruits and vegetables help to detoxify the body and reach a state of optimal health while we're being exposed to obesogens in our daily lives?

First, it's important to eat in a way that focuses on nutrient density while increasing the body's detoxification potential through the ingestion of antioxidants and botanicals. The body needs vitamins and minerals, as well as certain amounts of carbohydrates, fats and proteins. All of these elements are useless unless they can be efficiently absorbed into the body. Though many people are familiar with essential macro-minerals like iron and calcium, trace minerals are important co-factors found in the structure of certain enzymes and are indispensable in numerous biochemical pathways. It is enzymes that ultimately push the body to function properly and actively cleanse itself. The body's ability to self-cleanse is critical for true health and weight loss. Food can be metabolized more efficiently.

The keys to activating the body's natural cleansing programs are whole-body nutritional cleansing)as opposed to colon, liver or kidney cleansing) and ingesting the needed supply of trace minerals. Detoxifying the body is critical to healthy weight loss. It is the solution that delivers results that far surpassing of any popular conventional dieting program.

Chapter 5 ─────────
Personal Stories

The life-changing nutritional technology I am introducing to you is the reason I am still on this planet. But it is not just about me, it's what more than a million people have experienced by following the same program I have followed over the past decade.

There are so many stories of people who have had incredible life changing results with this new cleansing technology it is impossible to cover all but just a few of them. These stories may not be typical; however, they are their own personal stories that I have seen firsthand.

Dirck

My son's friend Dirck is in his mid-thirties and in relatively good shape, or so he thought.

He started on the nutritional cleanse and was amazed to release 19 ½ pounds. Although he was shocked, he thought it was remarkable, and so do I.

Linda

Another friend of mine had gained nearly 100 pounds **as a result of many medications**, and no matter what she did she could not get the excess weight off. I am happy to share that she has been able to release more than 50 pounds. Linda is well on her way to releasing those 100 pounds so much more quickly than any other diet or exercise program she had tried over the last 10 years.

Mark

This is Mark's story in his own words.

"For years, my doctor encouraged me to lose weight to improve my health and wellness, but I just wasn't ready to commit to downsizing my 500 plus-pound frame.

"Struggling from a lack of energy and spending long evenings in front of the TV, it wasn't until a close friend called me and told me about a new fat burning and nutritional cleansing family of products and a system from Isagenix that I began to consider the change. I researched the company, read testimonials, and talked to my wife before settling on trying the Cleansing and Fat Burning System.

"After using the system for 11 days, I felt more energized and I started to see weight coming off. I knew that this system was what I needed to get — and stay — motivated. With the support of my wife and grown children, family members and the friend who introduced me to the program and products, I made the decision to stick with the system for one year to see what I could accomplish.

"Now five years later and 388 pounds lighter and a charter member of the 300-Pound Club, it wasn't the numbers on the scale that kept me going; it was the milestones along the way.

"I knew from personal experience that if I stepped on a scale regularly and wasn't at my target weight that I'd think I wasn't successful. So, I set my goals on shirt, pant and belt sizes. I have since surpassed many of my previous targets, going from a size 64 pant to a size 32. It was just awesome when I went to a store to buy my first pair of Wranglers in 25 years, I had to bring them back and get a pair two sizes smaller.

"My all-time favorite milestone happened six months into my weight loss journey. I was walking through a store and my doctor walked right past me without noticing me. I just smiled and nodded. He came back after continuing to walk two aisles over and couldn't believe it was me; he didn't recognize me. It was one of the most gratifying moments.

"That is how my journey went and I hope by sharing it with those who have this kind of weight (or any amount of weight) will see what is possible. The most important thing is that I am maintaining my weight and my life has never been better.

"My total weight lost was 388 pounds and it has been maintained for five years since the journey began."

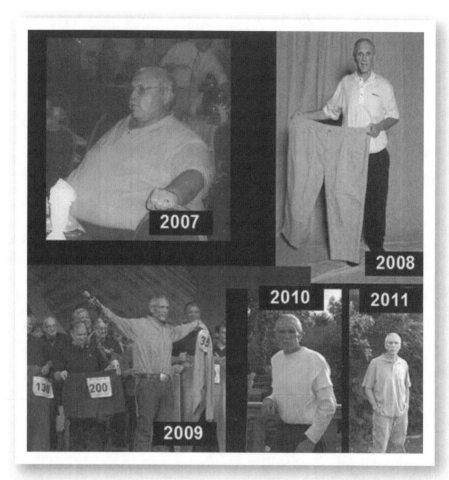

These amazing photographs show a glimpse of Mark's incredible journey. They have not been retouched or altered in any way. He transformed his body from a starting weight of 552 to 164 pounds and went from a size 64- to a 32-in. waist.

Drew and Colin

Before you think that the stories are only about weight loss I want to share one very close to my heart. It is the story of my two sons Drew and Colin. Drew, my oldest son, was a member of the University of Colorado ski team and in his early twenties when he tried this revolutionary cleanse. He did not think he needed to lose weight, but I assured him this was not exclusively a weight loss program.

Drew, like his friend Dirck, was shocked to release 15 pounds of fat and he said his energy was that of his teenage years. Drew has never missed a day on the program since.

My youngest son, Colin, was a 20-year-old all-state basketball player in great shape—or so he thought. He reluctantly went on the cleanse and quickly lost 10 pounds. Colin now never misses a day without being on these life-changing products.

Jill

"In the 3rd grade, my school nurse put me on the scale. She told me that I was fat and weighed more than she did. In that moment, at the tender age of 8, I felt ashamed of my weight.

"Fast forward 30 years, another moment when I was swimming with my family. My kids begged me to go down the pool slide. Before I knew it, I was wedged within the slide. As minutes passed, a family member worked on getting me out. Finally, out I came, mortified.

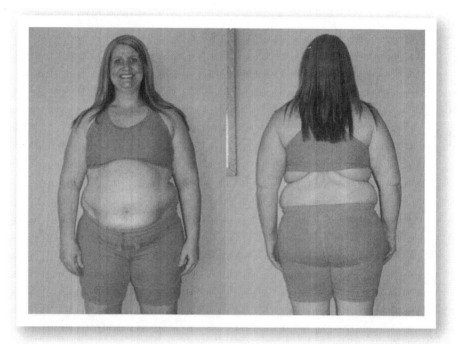

"Through the years, I've tried everything to lose weight, taking 'before' pictures 24 different times, each time saying to myself, 'this time I'll do it.' I failed every time, continuing my weight battle and food addictions.

"In April of 2010, I was desperate. I tried out for 'The Biggest Loser.' I became a semi-finalist, however, wasn't selected to appear on the show. I promised my close friend that if I wasn't selected, I would do Isagenix 'the right way.' With faith that God would help me conquer my addictions, I made good on my promise.

"My journey began the same time the Biggest Loser contestants went to their ranch. I made a Vision Board with the '100 Pound Club' as my main goal. I began slowly exercising and religiously following my eating plan. I was driven!"

"When the Biggest Loser finale aired, I'd achieved a higher percentage of weight loss than any of the female contestants.

"I've now released 131 pounds (half my body weight) and have gone from a size 22 to a size 4, which I also had on my Vision Board!

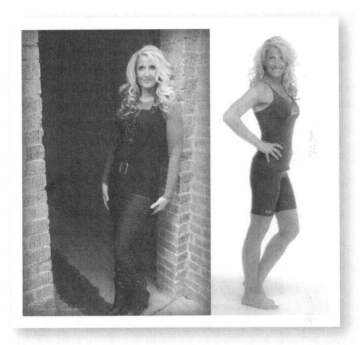

Jill lost 131 pounds!

"My new body has allowed me to accomplish things I never thought possible. For example, my son and I recently climbed to the top of a mountain near St. George. As we sat side by side on the summit, he turned to me with tears in his eyes and said, 'Mom, you did it. Thanks for getting healthy for us!' This was the same son who just a year before was embarrassed when I came to his school because someone told him he had a fat mom. Also, I recently ran three half marathon's, yet another goal on my Vision Board!

"With these priceless moments, I've realized that I will never again sit on the sidelines. I will live my healthy life to the fullest, achieving new milestones and creating new memories with my loved ones!

"I believe everyone should feel as exuberant as I do today! I've gained self-confidence and in return I'm helping thousands of people become the person God intended them to be."

Michael

Internationally renowned research scientist, Michael Colgan, Ph.D., C.C.N., discusses his own experience with the special whey in the Isagenix IsaLean® Shake and the triathletes who he trained. The following excerpts are from a lecture delivered by Dr. Colgan in 2010.

"In 1991, I wrote about this protein, this very protein now used by Isagenix. Before there was ever an IsaLean Shake, I wrote a book called *The Right Protein for Muscle and Strength.*

"And then when I came to Isagenix in May of 2010, the company John Anderson co-founded, I decided to study whether or not the system, the cleanse system, and the protein worked. Because there are many, many systems out there. There are hundreds of systems … I work with a lot of athletes. I was working with some triathletes, a group. I managed to persuade them … to do this nutritional cleanse for 30 days because they didn't want to lose muscle. They didn't want to reduce their food. They absolutely did not want to reduce their training. And then if their training was going to be reduced they were not going to do it… I joined this group myself because I wanted my own proof. I always want to have proof. Real solid stuff.

"So I did it on myself as well. And I started out at 8.95 body fat. And in 30 days I went down to 5.3% body fat. I hadn't seen my abs so well for 25 years.

"And all of the triathletes lost body fat. We lost an average of 4.9 pounds of body fat. Lost 3% of body fat. Do you think that their performance went down? No. Their performance went up. It's like taking a couple of bricks off your back."

William

My personal friend Dr. William Andrews is one of the leading geneticists in the world and has a Ph.D. in microbiology. Also, Dr. Andrews is a world-class, ultra-marathon runner. Ultra-marathon runners run in races of a minimum of 100 continuous miles. That is like running four normal marathons in a row, without stopping.

For years, Dr. Andrews has been researching nutrition to support his extraordinary athletic passion for marathon running, which he believes is important to living healthier and longer. But even though he exercised intensely, ate three healthy organic meals a day and didn't drink alcohol nor smoke cigarettes, he could not seem to lose the extra 15 pounds stored around his middle.

That was until I introduced him to the Isagenix system. Although Dr. Andrews was skeptical about the cleanse, it only took him 11 days to call me and say "Peter, what the heck is in this stuff?" Over the course of his first 11-day cleanse, he had a life-changing experience. Not only did he lose some of that stubborn weight, but he was amazed (and continues to be) at the improvement in his stamina and the increased speed in the ultra-marathons that he continues to run at 60 years of age. Dr. Andrews believes that this cleansing technology is the pathway to living healthier and longer and is the only anti-aging system available today.

In August 2012, Dr. Andrews completed one of the most grueling athletic challenges on earth—a 128 mile race through the Himalayas that included two of the world's highest mountain passes. Called "La Ultra—The High," this race is run at an average altitude of 14,765 ft. and reaches up to 17,700 ft. at its highest point. Competitors have to battle with an oxygen content that is approximately 66% less than at sea level. This race pushes human endurance to the limit and redefines human body and mind capabilities.

Dr. Andrews finished the race in 5th place with a time of 50 hours, 51 minutes, 52 seconds. This feat is amazing so many ways. His competitors ahead of him were half his age. Dr. Andrews is only one of 16 people in the world to complete the race.

Recently, Dr. Andrews lectured to a large group where he stated publicly that the Isagenix nutritional cleansing technology was a major reason he was able to compete at the highest level despite the fact that he is 60 years of age. Dr. Andrews has been consistently consuming the nutritional cleaning technology since July of 2010. As a world-class athlete, Dr. Andrews has access to any food and nutritional supplements on the planet. He said that there is nothing he has discovered that truly compares to this incredible nutritional cleansing technology. So, if you are an athlete and can find something better than this program, please let Dr. Andrews know.

Dr. Andrews consumes these nutritional cleansing products each and every day on a simple maintenance program. He has companies beating down his door to consume their products without charge, but instead he chooses to personally purchase this nutritional cleansing technology created by John Anderson.

Mike

When Mike started on Isagenix he weighed 366.2 pounds. He wore size 54 jeans and 5X t-shirt. His goal was to lose 230 pounds. He was 50 years old and lived alone when he started the program. Mike didn't get out much and his friends would find him sitting alone in his house in the dark when they would stop to visit him. He had to use a table or chair to help pull himself up from a sitting position. He said he sat around a lot because it was such a task just to walk from room to room.

Mike now weighs 235 pounds!

During his weight-loss process, Mike charted his blood pressure, pulse, and blood sugar. He also put himself on an exercise program that included riding an exercise bike and a road bike.

Mike said he surprised his doctor when he saw him some time after he started the program. He weighed 396 pounds the last time he saw his doctor. Now he weighed 294.8 pounds—more than100 pounds difference in weight! The doctor reviewed Mike's blood work and told him that his sugar levels were great, his cholesterol was normal and his blood pressure was good. He said Mike's magnesium and phosphorus and calcium levels were outstanding.

At this point, Mike was taking five different medications every day. Without the extra weight taking a toll on his body, Mike's doctor took him off four of his medications. He still takes thyroid medication.

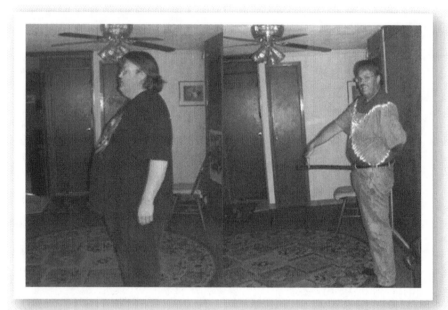

Now, Mike is active and gets out of the house regularly. He uses his exercise bike for 20 minutes every day and rides a road bike some-times twice a day for exercise. He is always doing projects during the day, whether it is working on other people's cars or projects around his house. Mike has a new lease on life. Not only does he have more energy to burn, but he says his appetite is satisfied. He also likes the fact that he doesn't crave food like he did before he started on Isagenix.

There are thousands of stories like these that show how you can lose weight, become healthier and live a longer, happier life.

Chapter 6

What We Need and What We Don't Need

Trace Minerals

The body must be supplied with proper nutrients for optimum functioning. One of the most important group of nutrients is ionic trace minerals. Ionic trace minerals are essential inorganic elements that are required in small amounts (less than 100 milligrams) for the normal physiologic processes of the body. The body requires ionic trace minerals and rare earth elements to speed up detox and antioxidant enzyme reactions in the body. For example, selenium is needed for the production of glutathione peroxidase, zinc is essential for many enzymes, cobalt is part of vitamin B_{12}, and is the vehicle that efficiently opens cells to receive and process nutrients.

Trace minerals support the majority of muscle function and are the key components for the performance of most body processes. While performing so many functions in the body, trace minerals also help eliminate our cravings for sugar and carbohydrates.

These little powerhouses have been called the spark plugs of life, so when they are lacking in the foods we eat, our ability to live life to the fullest is hindered. Imagine how your car would run if just one spark plug is not working. Ultimately, our human potential is dependent upon having sufficient trace minerals in our diet.

In today's society even if a food source is organically based, it may not contain the proper amount of trace minerals for optimal health, Our earth contains a balance of nutrients for us to be healthy. But after many years of aggressive farming, use of pesticides, and stripping off topsoil, we have depleted the essential nutrients in our crops. A report presented to the U.S. Senate describes how diet deficiencies are related to soil depletion. The soil in the U.S. had become almost void of minerals and our nation is suffering the health consequences. The catch is that the report was presented in 1936. If our food supply was nearly bankrupt of minerals 75 years ago, there is a good chance we have a worse situation today (Beach, 1936).

Trace minerals were one of the keys that transformed my life. Because of my eating habits, hey were either insufficient in my diet or lacking all together. It wasn't until I started using the nutrient-dense products formulated by John Anderson that I began really living again.

More than 30 years ago, John Anderson, who is considered the father of trace minerals, was awarded a patent on the extraction of trace ionic minerals from ancient plant deposits that were millions of years old. Called the "mineral man" for his extensive research and use of these trace minerals, Anderson was one of the pioneers in supplying trace minerals for human consumption.

Using his extensive knowledge of nutrients and trace minerals, John Anderson
founded Isagenix International in
March 2002 with Jim and Kathy
Coover, so he could develop and
manufacture high-quality systems for
cleansing, fat burning and nutrition.
From the first moment that I consumed John Anderson's nutritionally
dense Cleanse for Life® supplement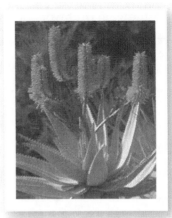
drink, I started replenishing the missing nutrients in my body and
reduced my frequent food cravings for sugar and simple carbohydrates. Furthermore, it was only when I started using this cleansing
technology that my body received appropriate quantities of these
life-changing elements.

This unique formulation contains aloe vera gel made from the inner
heart filet of aloe vera leaves that have been processed at low temperatures and spray dried to preserve the enzymes and nutrients.
The gel is where the leaf stores the majority of its nutrients, enzymes,
essential amino acids, vitamins and minerals, which support digestive health and the immune system while encouraging detoxification. Also, it is the inner filet that contains special polysaccharides,
which have been studied for their ability to balance the immune
system and their actions as natural detoxifiers, helping to move
along biochemical processes in the liver to neutralize toxins. Many
other aloe vera supplements use high heat that actually destroys the
polysaccharides and other nutrients.

In addition to the beneficial effects of aloe vera, the mineral supplement drink also includes bilberries, blueberries and raspberries, all of which serve as great sources of antioxidants, and are designed to work with all other nutrients to advance the cleansing processes.

Cleanse for Life® also fortifies me with more than 70 ionic trace minerals in a unique formulation from alfalfa, known as Ionic Alfalfa, to start me on the path to sustainable optimal health.

These nutritionally dense ingredients treat the body as a whole to relieve it of excess and nutritionally bankrupt waste. Now, my body performs the way it was designed, and self-regulates to achieve optimal health.

Essential Protein

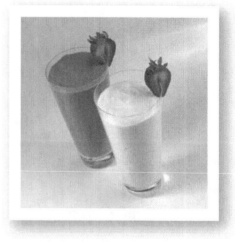

Half the dry weight of your body is protein—more than 100,000 different proteins. All of them have to be made from the proteins that you eat. If you eat inferior proteins you will grow an inferior body, no matter what else you do to guard your health. If you eat inferior proteins even for one day, they will grow into your body. You will then have to deal with them for the next six months, about the time that a muscle or organ cell lasts before replacement. If you eat that triple burger, it will grow into your muscles, your heart, and your brain.

To have a healthy body you have to get the right protein every day. Why? Because the human body does not store protein, but it does store fats and carbohydrates.

During my cleanse, I drank a whey protein-based meal supplement rich in essential branched-chain amino acids—called the IsaLean Shake—to satisfy my body faster and trigger muscle synthesis[1].

What is whey protein's critical role to our weight management, longevity, wellness—our very existence in the toxic world we live in today? The whey protein in these "super shakes" is in a class by itself when compared to other sources of protein like, meat, eggs, fish, soy and many other sources. The right whey protein has very unique properties, some of which mimic mother's breast milk—which is humanity's first perfect food.

IsaLean Shakes use extraordinary and uncommon New Zealand whey protein that can change the quality of your life and enhance your human potential and—specifically—your gene potential. Consuming these shakes provides me with incredible health benefits and energy that I am unable to get from other foods or protein sources.

These shakes mimic the ratio of whey protein and milk protein found in mother's breast milk which is 60% whey protein and 40% milk protein. Comparatively, regular cow's milk is 20% whey protein and 80% milk protein. In addition to whey protein, levels of milk protein are necessary while the body cleanses itself. These two milk proteins are both excellent sources of all the essential amino acids,

---

1 To learn more about these shakes, see Chapter 8—The Solution, Super Shakes at a Glance.

but they differ in one important aspect whey is a fast-digesting protein and milk protein is a slow-digesting protein. These keep amino acid levels in the blood steady over a longer period of time and promote optimal muscle growth (Dangin, M. et al, 2001).

I consumed protein shakes as an athlete all my life, and now I know that not all whey protein shakes are created equally. The whey protein found in this shake is derived from New Zealand dairy cows. In New Zealand, cattle are not treated with antibiotics or growth hormones, and their food sources are not riddled with herbicides and pesticides. In addition, the cows are only fed grass, not corn—which is a critical component as you will learn.

Glutathione

The amazing whey protein in the IsaLean Shakes is produced using a low-temperature, ultra-fine filtering process to keep the protein folds intact. In the United States, the majority of protein is processed using high-heat pasteurization that denatures protein, ultimately altering and destroying protein folds. Particularly, this high-heat process can compromise levels of cysteine, a crucial rate-limiting amino acid precursor needed to create a powerful antioxidant and major detoxification agent called glutathione. Glutathione is a substance that is critical for detoxification within the liver and in every cell in the body. Its production depends on the availability of several amino acids, along with available iron and an important trace mineral called selenium. This forms the enzyme glutathione peroxidase, which is a step in glutathione production and metabolism.

When glutathione production is low, detoxification in the liver is seriously impaired. This means the body is less able to eliminate all toxic metals, many toxic chemicals and other substances such as biological toxins (Wilson, 2011).

Glutathione is needed in every cell in the body to protect the cell membranes, cell proteins and DNA, and is one of two primary ways to detoxify the body. Most glutathione is produced naturally in the body, but the toxicity contained in most foods today destroys glutathione levels. There are supplements containing glutathione or glutathione-sparing nutrients; however, these nutritional supplements can be difficult for the body to absorb and will only provide minor benefits. Increasing glutathione launches the breakdown of impurities and allows my body to rid itself of toxins in a process known as "conjugation." The toxins attach to amino acids, allowing them to become water-soluble so they can be removed through the kidneys and liver.

Before starting this program, I had never heard of glutathione and now I understand why my health so dramatically improved with these nutritional cleansing technologies' amazing super calories and dense nutrition. The great news is that these unique IsaLean Shakes John Anderson created have all of the naturally occurring ingredients shown to significantly boost glutathione levels in the body.

Many of the thousands of research studies on glutathione have discovered that undenatured whey protein source is a great way to boost glutathione levels. The New Zealand whey protein in Isagenix's products is undenatured, which means that the protein folds haven't been altered by high heat or chemicals.

Research has also shown that the trace mineral selenium also plays a huge part in boosting glutathione levels. As you have learned, there are more than 70 trace minerals (including selenium) added to the shakes and all the other products that make up this nutritional cleansing technology.

Sarcopenia and What You Can Do About It

These shakes also include a high concentration of branched-chain amino acids, which not only help with the overall detoxification process in the body, but also maintain and build lean muscle to counteract an aging process known as sarcopenia—a process that contributes to the body's increased difficulty in holding onto muscle as it ages.

The body begins to lose about 1% of muscle mass per year after the age of 25, and this mass is often replaced with fat. Classic sarcopenia amounts to an approximate 40% loss of muscle mass between the ages of 25 and 70, resulting in frailty and drastic changes in metabolism. IsaLean Shakes combat this muscle loss by supplying the body with high levels of leuceine—a critical branched-chain amino acid linked with helping older individuals retain muscle and younger individuals double lean muscle development with exercise. My classic sarcopenia symptoms were eliminated within my own body and greatly altered my course of health for the rest of my life.

Sarcopenia is an age-related loss of skeletal muscle mass and function. According to Michael Colgan, Ph.D., who is considered one of the world's leading research scientists on protein for over 30 years, sarcopenia can be a deadly condition. He says, "Sarcopenia includes loss of muscle quantity and quality, loss of motor neurons that enable muscles to contract, loss of strength and especially muscle power, and a steep decline in muscle repair and recovery. Also, there is a progressive increase in oxidative stress, chronic inflammation, and pain."

Colgan says that muscles supply the immune system with the glutamine required to make immune cells, so when the body loses muscle it also loses immune function. Sarcopenia is also linked to death of brain cells and loss of cognition and memory with age because of reduced muscle contraction that leads to a decline of oxygen to the brain. He also notes that being overweight can mask the appearance of sarcopenia, which adds to the problem.

Sarcopenia was first measured accurately in 1989, and has grown to epidemic proportions in the U.S. and Canada. In otherwise healthy people over 40, it can be as high as one in every four tested. Colgan says that researchers on aging generally agree that it is a self-inflicted outcome that is almost 100% preventable (Colgan, 2001).

Colgan believes that sarcopenia is preventable by consuming sufficient high-quality protein to maintain lean muscle. Later in life it is most important to have the best quality protein possible, because synthesis of muscle protein becomes less efficient with age. Numerous studies, the latest just published in the *American Journal of Clinical Nutrition*, show that whey protein, similar to that found in IsaLean Shake, stimulates muscle protein uptake better than many other protein sources, including other shakes (Pennings, B. et al, 2011).

Research shows that for people over the age of 40, the recommended dietary allowance for protein (0.8 grams per kilogram) may not be sufficient. A controlled study found muscle was not maintained in subjects that ate the recommended daily allowances (Campbell, W. et al, 2001).

In additional to a high-quality whey protein meal supplement, it is important to include lactase and protease enzymes. Lactase breaks down the lactose, or milk sugar, found in many supplements, and protease breaks down proteins into peptides and amino acids to allow for greater absorption. With this in mind, John Anderson created the IsaLean Shake, which is the foundation of this nutritional cleansing technology. It is one of very few products on the market with lactase and protease that is a complete, low-calorie, nutritionally dense meal replacement.

Thermogenesis and Appetite

An important component to weight loss is thermogenesis. Thermogenesis occurs when a portion of dietary calories in excess of those required for immediate energy are converted to heat rather than stored as fat. When it comes to stimulating thermogenesis and satisfying appetite, it's well known that dietary protein is king over carbohydrates and fats. Now, a new study goes even further to show that the type of protein you choose is critical.

There are two major types of milk protein: casein (usually referred to as milk protein) and whey. According to research from the Nestle Research Center in Switzerland, whey protein consumed at breakfast, lunch and dinner proved most successful than either milk protein or soy proteins for boosting fat burning and simultaneously reducing muscle loss (Acheson, K. et al, 2011).

The scientists conducted a double-blind, randomized, placebo-controlled study, measuring the thermic effect of meals high in whey, milk protein or soy proteins, with a high carbohydrate meal as a control. They found that the total energy expenditure over 5.5 hours was greater after consuming the whey protein meal versus the other proteins. All were significantly higher than the high-carbohydrate meal (Acheson, K. et al, 2011).

The thermic effect of food is a measurement of the amount of energy that is required for digestion, absorption and metabolism. Put simply, the act of eating and digesting both brings in calories and burns them. Foods with a higher thermic effect can support weight management goals, while whey protein can promote muscle growth.

More than just a metabolic measure, the thermic effect of foods reflects the rate that fats, proteins and carbohydrates are broken down in our bodies for energy. The researchers explained the high thermic effect of whey protein might be due to its amino acid composition. Whey is high in leucine, a branched-chain amino acid, which has been shown to stimulate muscle protein synthesis and muscle maintenance.

In addition to boosting fat burning potential, a protein-rich diet also resulted in a much lower postprandial[2] glucose response than the carbohydrate control. We all know the feeling of an afternoon crash: eyes struggling to stay open, concentration drifting to thoughts of snuggling up in bed and overall energy depletion. Glucose may be the body's main fuel for energy, but now a new study suggests that

---

2 Occurring after a meal.

protein should be what we eat at lunch to help us stay awake and burn calories for the rest of the afternoon.

University of Cambridge researchers compared the effects of different nutrients on neurons in mouse brains. Wakefulness and calorie burning are dependent on secretion of a neuropeptide, orexin. When neurons don't secrete enough orexin, sleepiness ensues—which can lead to fewer calories burned and more weight gained over time. When the scientists measured the actions of protein (amino acids), carbohydrate (glucose), and fat (fatty acids) on the neurons, they found that the amino acids stimulated the cells to secrete orexin to a much greater extent than the other nutrients. In prior studies, the researchers found that orexin-secreting neurons are blocked by glucose. But when interactions between glucose and protein were looked at in this study, the researchers found that protein prevents glucose from blocking the orexin secretion. Lead researcher Denis Burdakov of the University of Cambridge Department of Pharmacology and Institute of Metabolic Science simply states, "Electrical impulses emitted by orexin cells stimulate wakefulness and tell the body to burn calories" (Karnani, M. et al, 2011).

This may help explain why people may feel particularly sleepy after eating meals rich in carbohydrates. Meals higher in protein and lower in total carbohydrates could help maintain alertness over the course of the day.

"What is exciting is to have a rational way to 'tune' select brain cells to be more or less active by deciding what food to eat. Not all brain cells are simply turned on by all nutrients, dietary composition is critical," says Burdakov.

For now, research suggests that if you have a choice between jam on toast or egg whites on toast, go for the latter! Even though the two may contain the same number of calories, having a bit of protein will tell the body to burn more calories out of those consumed (Karnani, M. et al, 2011).

Good and Bad Fats

Fats usually get a bad rap because many people aren't aware that there are both good and bad fats.

Fats from animal and vegetable sources provide a concentrated source of energy in the diet; they also provide the building blocks for cell membranes and a variety of hormones and hormone-like substances. As part of a meal fats slow down absorption, so we can go longer without feeling hungry. In addition, they act as carriers for the important fat-soluble vitamins A, D, E and K. Dietary fats are needed for the conversion of carotene to vitamin A, for mineral absorption and for a host of other processes. Many types of fats are critical for our bodies to function properly, but some fats are bad for us. In order to understand which ones, we must know something about the chemistry of fats.

Fats—or lipids—are a class of organic substances that are not soluble in water. Fatty acids are the building blocks of fats, much like amino acids are the building blocks of proteins. In simple terms, fatty acids are chains of carbon atoms with hydrogen atoms filling the available bonds. (Enig, M.; Fallon, S., 1999).

Fatty acids come in different chain lengths ranging from three carbon atoms long to 24 carbon atoms long. These fatty acids are either "saturated" (with an adequate number of hydrogen atoms) and chemically stable, or they are "unsaturated" (missing adequate hydrogen atoms) and chemically unstable. If a fatty acid is missing two hydrogen atoms, it is called a monounsaturated fatty acid, and in place of the two hydrogen atoms, the adjacent carbon atoms "double" bond to each other. If the fatty acid is missing four or six or more hydrogen atoms, it is called a polyunsaturated fatty acid, and it is even more unstable than the monounsaturated fatty acid. Because the double bonds in naturally occurring unsaturated fatty acids are curved with a "cis" configuration[3], the fatty acids cannot pack into a crystal form at normal temperatures, so their presence produces a liquid oil.

Saturated fatty acids have a straight configuration and pack together easily, so that they form a solid or semisolid fat at room temperature. This means that they do not normally go rancid, even when heated for cooking purposes. Our bodies make saturated fatty acids from carbohydrates, and they are found in animal fats and tropical oils.

---

3 Cis is the Latin term used in chemistry that means "on the same side." Cis configuration refers to unsaturated fatty acids that have hydrogen molecules on the same side of the carbon chain where there is a double bond.

Monounsaturated fatty acids have one double bond in the form of two carbon atoms double-bonded to each other and, therefore, lack two hydrogen atoms. Our bodies make monounsaturated fatty acids from saturated fatty acids and use them in a number of ways. Monounsaturated fats have a kink or bend at the position of the double bond, so they do not pack together as easily as saturated fats and, therefore, tend to be liquid at room temperature. Like saturated fats, they are relatively stable. They do not go rancid easily and can be used in cooking. The monounsaturated fatty acid most commonly found in our food is oleic acid, the main component of olive oil, as well as the oils from almonds, pecans, cashews and avocados.

Polyunsaturated fatty acids have two or more pairs of double bonds and, therefore, lack four or more hydrogen atoms. The two polyunsaturated fatty acids found most frequently in our foods are double unsaturated linoleic acid, with two double bonds—also called omega-6; and triple unsaturated linolenic acid, with three double bonds—also called omega-3. Our bodies cannot make these fatty acids, which is why they are called "essential." We must obtain our essential fatty acids or EFAs from the foods we eat. The polyunsaturated fatty acids have kinks or turns at the position of the double bond and hence do not pack together easily. They are liquid, even when refrigerated. The unpaired electrons at the double bonds make these oils highly reactive. They go rancid easily—particularly omega-3 linolenic acid—and must be treated with care. Polyunsaturated oils should never be heated or used in cooking. In nature, the polyunsaturated fatty acids are usually found in the cis form, which means that both hydrogen atoms at the double bond are on the same side.

Omega-6

Problems associated with an excess of polyunsaturates are exacerbated by the fact that most polyunsaturates in commercial vegetable oils are in the form of double unsaturated omega-6 linoleic acid, with very little of vital triple unsaturated omega-3 linolenic acid. Recent research has revealed that too much omega-6 in the diet creates an imbalance that can interfere with production of important prostaglandins (Lasserre, M. et al, 1985). This disruption can result in increased tendency to form blood clots, inflammation, high blood pressure, irritation of the digestive tract, depressed immune function, sterility, cell proliferation, cancer and weight gain (Fallon, S., 1996).

Omega-3

A number of researchers have argued that along with a surfeit of omega-6 fatty acids, the American diet is deficient in the more unsaturated omega-3 linolenic acid. This fatty acid is necessary for cell oxidation, for metabolizing important sulphur-containing amino acids and for maintaining proper balance in prostaglandin production. Most commercial vegetable oils contain very little omega-3 linolenic acid and large amounts of the omega-6 linoleic acid. In addition, modern agricultural and industrial practices have reduced the amount of omega-3 fatty acids in commercially available vegetables, eggs, fish and meat. For example, organic eggs from hens allowed to feed on insects and green plants can contain omega-6 and omega-3 fatty acids in the beneficial ratio of approximately one-to-one; but commercial supermarket eggs can contain as much as nineteen times more omega-6 than omega-3!

Trans Fats

Hydrogenation is the process that turns polyunsaturates, normally liquid at room temperature, into fats that are solid at room temperature— these fats are generally used in margarine and shortening. This is the process that creates trans fats. To produce them, manufacturers begin with the cheapest oils—soy, corn, cottonseed or canola, which are already rancid from the extraction process. Then they mix them with tiny metal particles—usually nickel oxide. The oil with its nickel catalyst is then subjected to hydrogen gas in a high-pressure, high-temperature reactor. To give it a better consistency, soap-like emulsifiers and starch are squeezed into the mixture and then the oil is again subjected to high temperatures when it is steam-cleaned. This removes its unpleasant odor due to rancidity. Margarine's natural color, an unappetizing grey, is removed by bleach. Dyes and strong flavors must then be added to make it resemble butter.

When unsaturated fatty acids are altered by hydrogenation, their curved cis configuration is straightened when one hydrogen atom of the pair is moved to the other side so that the molecule has some of the physical packing properties of saturated fatty acids. This is called the trans[4] formation, rarely found in nature. It is this process that changes a mostly unsaturated oil into a solid fat. The trans fatty acids are the same length and weight as the original cis fatty acid they were formed from, and although they have the same number of carbons, hydrogens,and oxygens, they are shaped differently. The problem arises when trans fatty acids are consumed from foods and they are deposited in those parts of the cell membranes that are supposed to have either saturated fatty acids or cis unsaturated fatty acids; under these circumstances the trans fatty acids essentially disrupt essential functions in the body (Enig, 2000).

---

4 Trans means "across or other side," so trans fatty acid means that the carbon chain has a pair of hydrogen atoms on opposite sides linked by a double bond.

Most of these manmade trans fats are toxins to the body. Altered hydrogenated fats made from vegetable oils actually block utilization of essential fatty acids, causing many deleterious effects including sexual dysfunction, increased blood cholesterol and paralysis of the immune system. Consumption of hydrogenated fats is associated with a host of other serious diseases, not only cancer but also atherosclerosis, diabetes, obesity, immune system dysfunction, low-birth-weight babies, birth defects, decreased visual acuity, sterility, difficulty in lactation and problems with bones and tendons (Enig, M., 1995).

Dr. Dennis Harper says, "Fatty foods have been maligned for many years and not for the right reasons. Most people seem to lump all fats together as though they were the same evil food that we should all avoid."

He also says that if we consume trans fats and our body uses them to create new cells, these new cells will leak, which will cause the cells to die. When cells die they can produce lipid peroxidation which can age the body prematurely.

The only problem with healthy fats that are found in nature would be if they have been contaminated by pesticides, hormones, heavy metals or other toxic substances. If they have been contaminated, these toxins reside in the fats and could cause cellular death in the body. For this reason, it is important to eat clean food. This generally means organic, if you can find it, or growing or raising it yourself, according to Dr. Harper.

Including good fats that are toxin-free into your cleanse is much like starting a campfire. At first, only a little bit of tinder is needed for the spark to catch fire. As time goes on, the tinder burns faster. Larger logs are needed for the fire to steadily burn. Similarly, fats are necessary in some quantities if you want to continue the fat-burning processes for an extended length of time.

So, low fat diets are not what they are purported to be at all. The body needs good fats for many of its functions like making and supporting ligaments and tendons.

In the book *Why Women Need Fat*, authors William D. Lassek, M.D., and Steven J.C. Gaulin Ph.D. explain why so much of what we have been taught about food and diets by nutritional experts—and especially our government—is false and misleading. The authors emphasize that the National Dietary Guidelines and its "food pyramid" claims that fat—especially saturated fat—is supposed to be bad for us, while polyunsaturated fat is thought to be better are not supported by credible studies. None that show reducing total and saturated fat while increasing polyunsaturated fat will make us healthier.

According to the authors, one review analyzed 21 different studies and concluded that there was no evidence that saturated fat in the diet increases the risk of heart attacks or strokes. (Lassek, W.; Gaulin, S., 2012) Another review found a complete lack of scientific evidence supporting any of the current recommendations in the U.S. Dietary Guidelines[5]. In fact, no large-scale study has ever shown that changing fat in the diet in accordance with Dietary Goals lowers the death rate or extends life. They maintain that the American people began to increase our weight at the same time we began making changes in our national diet. These changes occurred because of flawed high-profile studies conducted by Ancel Keys[6] and other researchers, who disregarded results that didn't coincide with their beliefs.

Because of these flawed studies, Americans started reducing saturated fat in our diets. How did this change affect us? According to

---

5 Beginning in 1980, the U.S. Department of Agriculture and Department of Health and Human Services has published an updated Dietary Guidelines for Americans. The most recent one, published in December 2010, recommends reducing saturated fat intake to 7% of caloric intake, down from its previously recommended 10%.

6 Ancel Keys, the father of K-rations for the military, published a study in 1953 that correlated deaths from heart disease with the percentage of calories from fat in the diet. He found that fat consumption was associated with an increased rate of death from heart disease in the six countries that he studied. He followed this up with a more detailed Seven Country Study published in 1970. This study led to the McGovern Report and the U.S. Dietary Guidelines. In his Six Country Study, Ancel Keys ignored data available from 16 other countries that did not fall in line with his desired graph. He did the same thing with his Seven Country Study by not using data from all 22 countries. If he had used data from these other countries he could have shown that increasing the percentage of calories from fat in the diet reduces the number of deaths from coronary heart disease.

Lassek and Gaulin, "during the thirty years that the calorie share of fat in our diets was going down, our weights were going sharply up." Looking at the evidence, there is little to suggest that fat intake is related to weight.

Lassek and Gaulin believe that the most important change in the American diet over the past forty years has been a huge increase in the consumption of vegetable oils that are high in polyunsaturated fat. More than three-quarters of this vegetable oil is soybean oil (nearly 500 calories a day), which is seven times more soybean oil consumed than in the European diet and much more than any other country in the world. Most of the rest of the oil we consume is corn oil, and we eat five times more of this than Europeans. According to Lassek and Gaulin, our appetite for soybean oil and corn directly correlates with American's historical weight gain. They say that soybean and corn oils promote weight gain because of the very large amounts of polyunsaturated omega-6 linoleic acid that they contain.

The authors go on to say that, "more than half of the vegetable oil we consume is polyunsaturated fat, mostly omega-6 linoleic acid, the same kind of fat that was mistakenly believed to lower our cholesterol. The amount of polyunsaturated omega-6 fat in our diet has more than doubled and now supplies more than 10% of our calories. We do need some omega-6, but a diet this high in omega-6 linoleic acid is unprecedented in human existence and extremely unnatural" (Lassek, W.; Gaulin, S., 2012).

At the turn of the century, most of the fatty acids in the diet were either saturated or monounsaturated, primarily from butter, lard, tallows, coconut oil and small amounts of olive oil. Today most of the fats in our diet are polyunsaturated from vegetable oils derived mostly from soy, as well as from corn, safflower and canola.

Modern diets can contain as much as 30% of calories as polyunsaturated oils, but scientific research indicates that this amount is far too high. The best evidence indicates that our intake of polyunsaturates should not be much greater than 4% of our caloric total intake (Lasserre, M. et al, 1985).

Excess consumption of polyunsaturated oils has been shown to contribute to a large number of disease conditions including increased cancer and heart disease (Felton, C. et al, 1994); immune system dysfunction; damage to the liver, reproductive organs and lungs; digestive disorders; depressed learning ability (Pinckney, E. et al, 1973); impaired growth; and weight gain (Valero-Garrido, D. et al, 1990).

In addition, it is now clear that polyunsaturated oils lower our good cholesterol or HDL. Lassek and Gaulin say, "the enormous and unnatural increase in industrially produced soybean and corn oils in the American diet is what has made us fatter. In 165 countries around the world, women weigh more where there is more corn and soybean oil in the diet" (Lassek, W.; Gaulin, S., 2012).

To back up their claims, Lassek and Gaulin discuss a study conducted in the late 1990s where researchers in Heidelberg, Germany studied dietary fat and weight gain in 11,000 women aged thirty-five and older for six years. The study shows that the most important single dietary factor related to women's weight gain was the amount of omega-6 linoleic acid in their diet.

Omega-6 linoleic acid itself does not appear to have any function in our bodies, but it is converted into arachidonic acid. This type of omega-6 linoleic acid produces molecules called eicosanoids. Eicosanoids that are made from arachidonic acid promote the growth and development of fatty tissue and fat storage and increase inflammation. In contrast, omega-3 fats produce a type of eicosanoid that decreases fat storage and decreases inflammation, according to Lassek and Gaulin.

Omega-6 fats also play a role in creating endocannabinoids in our bodies, which are natural brain compounds similar to THC—the active ingredient in marijuana. Endocannabinoids are known to play a role in numerous physiological processes, including appetite stimulation, memory and pain (National Institutes of Health, 2009). According to a study in 2011, a diet that is high in omega-6 polyunsaturated fatty acids will cause an increase in endocannabinoid signaling system activation and stimulate tissue specific activities that decrease insulin sensitivity in muscle and promote fat accumulation in the adipose tissue (Kim,J; Li, Y; Watkins, B, 2011).

The other way the omega-6 in our diet makes us gain weight is by decreasing omega-3 in our bodies—the fat that helps make us thinner. In the German study of dietary fat and weight gain, the more omega-3 fats in a woman's diet (alpha-linolenic, DHA, and EPA) the less weight she gained over time (Lassek, W.; Gaulin, S., 2012).

Instead of increasing fat storage and weight gain, omega-3 helps to reduce weight by increasing fat burning and decreasing the amount of fat we store. Also, omega-3 helps decrease our appetite. It is common to be more hungry after meals high in omega-6 linoleic acid and less hungry after meals high in omega-3. Omega-3 fats also help improve the way our cells respond to insulin, which can improve blood sugar control.

Lassek and Gaulin say that in 1960 we consumed nine times more omega-6 than omega-3, while today we have more than 21 times as much. Making matters worse, we have also been getting less omega-3 (EPA and DHA) from some of the natural sources—meat, poultry, eggs and fish.

"The amount of omega fats in meat depends on what the animals eat. And most animals are now fed corn instead of grass because it's cheaper. Since corn is much higher in omega-6 and much lower in omega-3 than grass, the change in animal feeds has lowered the omega-3 in meat and eggs while increasing omega-6. Also, while chicken meat and eggs still have some omega-3 EPA and DHA they now have much more omega-6 than omega-3 because chickens have also been switched over to corn-based feed" (Lassek, W.; Gaulin, S., 2012). That is why it is so significant that IsaLean Shakes are made with whey protein from cows that only eat grass.

Dr. Donald Miller, a cardiac surgeon and professor of surgery at the University of Washington School of Medicine in Seattle, puts our nation's health crisis in perspective. He says that 100 years ago less than one in 100 Americans were obese and coronary heart disease was unknown. Pneumonia, diarrhea, enteritis and tuberculosis were the most common causes of death. Now, a century later, the two most common causes of death are coronary heart disease and cancer, which account for 75% of all deaths. There were 500 cardiologists practicing in the U.S. in 1950. There are 30,000 of them now—a

60-fold increase for a population that has only doubled since 1950 (Miller, D., 2011).

He goes on to say that an epidemic of obesity has accompanied the adoption of a low-fat diet. With only 1 in 150 people obese when the century began, by 1950 nearly 10% of Americans were obese. Thirty years later, in 1980, it had risen to 15%. Then following publication of the U.S. Dietary Guidelines and its every-five-year updates, obesity in Americans has steadily risen. Now, two-third of the American public is overweight and more than one-third is obese. Today the average American weighs 30 pounds more that he or she did 100 years ago. American women weigh an average of 167 pounds and men weigh and average of 191 pounds.

Dr. Miller contends that, "there is solid evidence that this epidemic of obesity has resulted from replacing saturated fat in the American diet with carbohydrates and processed polyunsaturated vegetable oils" (Miller, D., 2011).

These are some of the reasons why we have become one of the most overfed and undernourished societies on earth. Look around at our obese nation. Is the Food Pyramid working? We have been flat out misled at the very least. There was never any evidence that saturated fats were bad; it is the polyunsaturated omega-6 fats that are bad while the omega-3 fats are good. Armed with this important knowledge, we can find a solution to our giant obesity problem and end the diets that fail us.

Chapter 7
The Solution

The Healing Practice of Cleansing

Cleansing has been a traditional healing practice to enhance many of the body's internal detoxification and cleansing systems for thousands of years. Throughout history, a common method for cleansing has been fasting, a method in which only a combination of herbal teas or special botanicals are ingested. Reduced food intake allows the body to purify itself through rest and renewal, while botanicals—such as aloe gel, licorice root and ashwagandha root—contain bio-active components to support the liver (the body's natural detoxifier) and individual cells.

Age-old traditions of cleansing have now been combined with modern technologies to create dietary supplements that provide nourishment that deal efficiently with daily toxic loads and stresses. In my own quest to detoxify my body, I used the Isagenix Cleanse for Life®—a drink specialized to support the liver, immune system and overall cellular health by utilizing a combination of vitamins, herbal teas and other botanical ingredients.

The ingredients chosen for the Cleanse for Life® drink help protect my body from daily pollutants and promoted a state of "deep cleansing," which I have found to be a sound approach to weight management.

This nutritional cleansing technology was introduced to the world in 2002 by Isagenix, the world leader in whole-body nutritional cleansing, cellular replenishing and youthful aging. This groundbreaking cleansing technology was invented by John Anderson who has formulated and manufactured more than 2,500 nutritional formulations for more than 600 companies.

Anderson proved the results of this technology by taking on a life-threatening health challenge and being the first person to ever use the Isagenix cleansing and fat-burning technology. He experienced tremendous, fast and safe weight loss while guarding against lean muscle loss. He also worked with doctors and health professionals to pinpoint how and why the program worked so well in comparison to other diet approaches. His innovative discovery has changed nutritional science and helped improve the lives of countless people.

As a result, Anderson is optimistic about the future. He states, "I believe this year, 2012, is the beginning of the next generation of nutrition. We'll see more discoveries over the next five years than anyone can imagine. My continued involvement in nutraceutical research sciences today is the most important time of my life and has made more progress in the last 24 months than in the past 30 years combined. Where will we be next year? You will see miracles and fiction become a reality."

Balanced nutrition and nutritional cleansing are key strategies for coping with daily toxins, but there are others. Since there's no way to avoid all toxins, and balanced nutrition and nutritional cleansing are only partial strategies for coping, additional measures must be taken. The goal, of course, is to reduce toxic exposure as much as possible. I was able to achieve this by making simple lifestyle changes, such as choosing fruits and vegetables free of pesticides, drinking more water, using non-toxic skin care products and being in the fresh air whenever possible.

How Does the Program Work?

The following cleansing program is not a diet that focuses on counting calories, but a complete program that allows the body to cleanse itself.

It all begins with a 9-day nutritional cleanse[1], plus two pre-cleanse days. It also includes deep cleansing days and shake days, which I will describe in more detail.

During my cleanse, it surprised me that even on deep cleanse days when I was only ingesting liquid nutrition, my body was fed and satisfied with massive amounts of liquid nutrition, and though caloric intake is severely reduced, the body is not denied the important nutrients and trace-minerals it needs. I was pleasantly surprised that I was not hungry.

As my body was optimally supplied with the necessary nutrients without all the calories, my body naturally began to cleanse itself

---

1 For more information see Appendix II - Sample Chart: 9-Day Cleanse and 2-Day Pre-Cleanse.

by utilizing the massive amounts of these nutrients contained in the four products that made up this life-changing cleansing technology.

The trace-minerals supported the enzymes that naturally occur in my body. Impurities stored in fat cells traveled to my liver to be detoxified. The liver then released these impurities as bile or converted them into water-soluble waste to be processed by my liver and excreted from my body through the colon. This process differs from a colon cleanse, which is designed to release toxins only in the colon, not the toxins stored in our fat cells.

While I was on the Isagenix cleanse, I consumed IsaLean-Shakes and a series of chewable nutritional snacks (also created by John Anderson) that are packed with the same New Zealand whey protein that is in the IsaLean Shakes. These low-calorie snacks helped to curb my hunger by providing small amounts of proteins, fats and carbohydrates throughout the day, which kept my body in balance and prevented an "afternoon crash" of energy. These snacks maintained overall balance in my body. The proteins supported lean muscle development, the carbohydrates broke down into glucose, keeps my brain sharp, and the ionic trace-minerals kept me fully nourished.

These nutritionally dense snacks contain organic coconut oil, which is needed to slow down the release of glucose, maintain my body's fat-burning processes and stimulate metabolism firings.

The last component in the cleanse is what I like to refer to as a super vitamin. John Anderson also formulated this super vitamin or unique capsule—called the Natural Accelerator—to assist my body in burning fat without the use of stimulants. These capsules naturally invigorate my body to maintain energy throughout the day while on the cleanse. Each capsule contains Ionic Alfalfa trace minerals and a variety of natural ingredients, including apple cider vinegar, green tea leaf extract, niacin, cinnamon-dried bark and cayenne pepper.

These natural nutrients ensure that my body is constantly satisfied with pure nourishment, even though I eat a low-calorie diet. (Keep in mind that the Natural Accelerator is for appetite support and not for appetite suppression.)

Why Does the Cleanse Produce Such Dramatic Results?

Herein lies the secret to the long-lasting success of this revolutionary nutritional cleanse: though low in calories, the Isagenix nutritional cleanse provided me with nutritionally dense calories.

As I have previously discussed, most of today's foods are not nutritionally balanced or nutritionally dense, so people continue to crave and consume more and more food that never fully nourishes or satisfies them. However, the Isagenix cleansing technology supplies massive amounts of nutrition, along with critical ionic trace minerals, in very few calories. The cleanse supplies the body with many more nutrients than the minimum 51 we require for minimum body functions.

During my cleansing experience, antioxidant botanicals such as aloe gel, licorice root and ashwagandha root supported liver detoxification and reduced my cravings. My body was consistently and sufficiently nourished with nutritious elements and ionic trace minerals instead of empty calories.

Even when my body was immersed in a deep cleanse day, I was continually satisfied because for the first time I was supplied with the appropriate amounts of nutrition and ionic trace minerals—a need that extends far beyond just calories. Having done the research, I now know why I was satisfied by the nutritional density. It had nothing to do with the amount of calories I was ingesting.

This is a new paradigm in nutritional science. After enlisting in this program, it forever changed my perceptions of the true meaning of health. I now know it is not the number of calories that matter in achieving a healthy lifestyle, but the make-up of nutrition that is contained within the calories.

Phil, the friend of mine who lost almost 200 pounds, was astonished at the weight he released. Not only was he not hungry, but he completely changed his eating habits because his cravings diminished almost overnight. This is not magic; it is really happening to more than a million people.

Researchers and scientists are beginning to recognize the new paradigm for food, nutrition and wellness—it has to be about nutrition and not calories. That is why people are achieving extraordinary results on the cleanse. Like my friend, Mark, who was full and satisfied even though he was eating a fraction of the calories he thought he needed to survive when he was nearly 600 pounds No matter how many empty calories he consumed, he was still satisfied. Those foods were devoid of all the 51 nutrients necessary to satisfy his body. Will power cannot work if your body is struggling with hunger because it does not have the nutrition it needs. This nutritional cleanse has many more than 51 of the essential nutrients.

Imagine that a new gasoline additive was invented that allowed cars to get 100 or 200 miles per gallon instead of approximately 20 miles per gallon. The same concept lies behind the nutritional super calorie. Just as the car would use much less gasoline and still travel much farther, this nutritional cleansing technology provides the body with significantly more nutrients in fewer calories. The body is able to function much more efficiently.

For me, the cleansing approach is far beyond a weight loss program. By introducing me to these extraordinarily dense foods (and the super-nutritional calories they contain, I was catapulted into a lifestyle of full wellness. I now have more energy, sharpened mental clarity and a new zest for life—benefits that were just as significant as the weight loss I achieved. Nutritional cleansing has set me on a path toward youthful aging, longevity and a maximization of my personal human potential. I've achieved a state of well-being that keeps me energized and engaged constantly in my daily life. It allows me for the first time in my life to achieve two critical goals: First and foremost, to live healthier and longer; second, to maximize my human potential. Along with my increased energy and improved mental clarity, I have lower stress and boundless energy, and I sleep like a baby. These are just a few of the benefits I have experienced. As a result, I am maximizing my human potential.

This is why this program is so much more than a weight-loss strategy. I hear story after story about how people are getting so much more out of cleansing than just the weight loss and, perhaps more importantly, the fat they are releasing. Recently, I got a call from a woman named Sharon, who had been on the cleanse for six days. She said she is amazed at the amount of energy she has and she can't believe how well she is sleeping. Although she started the program because she wanted to lose weight, she now says the energy and the deep sleep she gets far surpass the weight she is releasing. My personal trainer told me just last week that he cannot believe how this has helped him reduce his overall body fat percentage, increased his flexibility and reduced his recovery time after workouts. This is a young man who is in incredible shape, and he has enhanced and improved his performance. Although he was skeptical at first, now he says this is the only protein and cleansing program he will ever use and recommend to his clients. These stories are so common now that I have just included a few to give you an overall picture of what you might experience. I hope you have as great as an experience as the ones I've talked about here.

What Is a Pre-Cleanse Day?

The two pre-cleanse days at the beginning of the program prepare the body to truly take advantage of the deep cleanse days. My body began to burn fat even during the pre-cleanse period, as I cut out unnecessary elements of my daily diet, such as caffeine, sugars, diet sodas and alcohol. I only drank an IsaLean Shake for breakfast and dinner, and ate a healthy 400-600 calorie meal of my choice for lunch.

During this time, I began consuming a minimum of eight 8-oz. glasses of water each day. In order to get the most out of my cleansing experience, I drank half my body weight in number of ounces of water a day. Water is an integral part of any cleansing program, and drinking the necessary amount of water daily is an important habit in order to maintain smooth functioning within the body. This does not mean that water can be replaced with the small amounts contained in tea or soda. Pure water is the lifeblood of the body and a main vehicle for carrying nutrients. It also disposes of the body's waste and facilitates detoxification processes.

Every day through urination, perspiration and respiration, we lose the equivalent of at least eight 8-oz. glasses of water. In order to replenish this supply we must drink substantial amounts of clean, purified water.

Deep Cleansing

After increasing my water intake and familiarizing my body with cleansing nutrients during the pre-cleanse days, I began two days of the deep cleanse. In the Isagenix program, all deep cleansing days are the same: solid food is replaced with aloe vera-based liquid nutrition in the Cleanse for Life® drink, whey protein snacks and a Natural Accelerator capsule.

In the first 24 hours of deep cleansing—while solid food was not consumed—my body used up the sugar and glycogen stored in my liver and began producing growth hormones to trigger fat burning and support lean muscle mass.

On the first day of the deep cleanse, I consumed four ounces of the aloe vera nutrients four times a day, six to eight of the nutritional

Isagenix snacks and two Natural Accelerator capsules. Because these supplements flooded my body with massive amounts of nutrients, trace-minerals, fats and proteins, I didn't experience hunger, even without solid foods.

Though the body begins its fat-burning processes on the first deep cleanse day, by the end of the second day, excess sugar and carbohydrates stored in the liver have been used up and 100% fat burning has been achieved.

Within just the first 24 hours of deep cleansing, the body burns excess glycogen (stored sugar). During the second 24 hours it begins to turn to fat energy—the very fat in which the impurities are stored. The body begins to burn off this excess fat, causing the body to shed pounds and inches quickly and safely. Throughout the cleanse, the body continues to increase levels of growth hormone to build muscle as the fat was released.

For me, the first two days of the deep cleanse really showed in how well my formerly too-tight jeans fit. Was this possible? In such a short period of time I was shrinking.

After the first round of deep cleanse days, I completed five days of replenishment, so my body could rest and prepare for another round of serious cleansing. By the morning of the fifth day, I was amazed at how many inches I was shedding and how much energy I had. It astounded me that this cleansing technology was already changing my world. And, after drinking half or nearly half of my body weight in number of ounces of water daily, I realized there was no way this weight loss could be explained away as just a loss of "water weight."

On the fifth day, I returned to a shake for breakfast, a single healthy meal at lunch, and another shake for dinner, along with a combination of Isagenix super vitamins and snacks. The shakes provided the perfect combinations of carbohydrates, fats, proteins and Ionic Alfalfa to continue the fat burning and self-cleansing processes. I continued this routine through the ninth day. I returned to a state of deep cleansing on the tenth and eleventh days, and my body resumed intense fat burning. These days were great opportunities for my body to really "clean house" of the remaining toxins, so I could achieve optimal health and weight loss.

By following all recommendations in this program, my body's processes continued efficiently and effectively, undisturbed by my major dietary changes.

Other friends said they had no weight to lose at all did the cleanse, and they were shocked to drop pounds they did not think they had to lose. Of course, it was their bodies shedding this extraneous fat that was only there to store impurities. As the body began to cleanse itself, it let go of this extra fat. This nutritional cleanse has so many people scratching their heads and saying, "I cannot believe my scale." That is because they are used to conventional dieting, which simply does not and cannot produce such life-changing results in such a short time period safely. This is revolutionary and can, in fact, transform your beliefs about diet, exercise and your human potential.

Although results may vary, people are astounded at these common results. Many traditional dieters are excited if they can lose a pound a week. By constantly replenishing any water flushed out of our bodies during the cleanse, this was guaranteed not to be a mere water weight loss that will be gained back right away. Knowing we could achieve our weight goals so quickly and safely motivated me and many other people to continue the program.

Race to Maintenance Program

What do you do once you complete the cleanse if you have more weight to lose, like Mark Webber and myself? Or, you feel so good you want to cleanse some more until you feel more satisfied?

To meet this demand, Dr. Dennis Harper and I developed the "Race to Maintenance[2]" program because, for many who have just completed the cleanse, their bodies risk abandoning full fat-burning mode if they choose to immediately return to their old eating habits. Thousands have experienced a rapid completion to their goals. The schedule is an easy guide for you to follow on a daily basis.

A free cleansing coach is also available during this period to assist and ensure that you follow program correctly so that achieve the best possible results. As the name implies, the Race to Maintenance is to get you to a maintenance program with the least amount of effort in the shortest period of time possible. Your body will thank you and reward you with living healthier and longer.

To maintain the same high fat-burning intensity after cleansing, the body now requires more fuel. Unlike most conventional diets, this requires an increase in calories, while continuing to infuse the body with the massive amounts of nutrients and traceminerals. My

---

2 For more information see Appendix III - Sample Chart: Race to Maintenance.

"Race to Maintenance" program begins on day 12 and continues for five days. I have a shake for breakfast, a healthy lunch, a healthy dinner and a shake for dessert. These five days are "feast days" that include regular meals with the family as well as shakes. Unlike a diet, this program actually increases the daily caloric intake with nutrient dense calories. These days are followed by two days of deep cleansing for a total 7-day cleanse. I repeat this 7-day cycle for three consecutive weeks for a total of 21 days. This, in addition to the first 9-day cleanse, puts my body on a nutritional cleanse course for a full month.

During the "Race to Maintenance" period, it is important that the IsaLean Shake be the final meal of the day to supply the body with that special blend of enzymes, nutrients and trace minerals for continued fat burning. Since the amount of solid food is reduced on these days, the body's rate of fat burning and its basal metabolic rate—the rate at which calories are burned when the body is at rest—are slowed, and you may experience a plateau in weight loss. However, drinking the shake keeps carbohydrates down, so they don't interfere with the human growth hormone production and will ensure sustained fat burning.

If you want to lose more weight after the month, you can continue on the 7-day Race to Maintenance rotation until your target weight is reached. Back-to-back cleansing will position the body in a longer state of fat burning that cannot be fully achieved in the initial 11-day cleanse.

Even with a lot of weight to lose, many people find they are able to maintain this dietary cycle until they reach their goals. As long as they are careful to consume calories comprised of no more than 40% carbohydrates and eat no more than 600 calories per meal, their bodies are properly fueled to continue burning fat. As they continue to feel better and become more nourished and active, the new life they achieve motivates them throughout the process.

I spoke to a recent cleansing participant in his mid-thirties who really had very little weight to lose. His name is Will and he only lost a few pounds, as that was all he needed to lose. He says, "I cannot believe the amount of energy that I have. It is not speed energy; it is natural and long lasting."

Another participant who is a sales manager in a high stress job said she is waking up at 6 a.m. and jumping out of bed. She said before the cleanse she dreaded mornings and now she has to make herself sleep in until 6 a.m. She is amazed that all day long she has energy and is not getting the cravings during the midday that she used to get. She says, "Many days I have to remind myself to eat lunch as I am so satisfied. You could have never convinced me there could be such an amazing food. It is wonderful to feel so full of energy and vitality."

My good friend, Charlie, started at 414 pounds and has released an astounding 42 pounds utilizing the Race to Maintenance program after his cleanses. He cannot believe that he is not hungry. He failed on all the previous diets he tried because he always felt hungry. On the Race to Maintenance he is able to stick to it. My other friend, Fred, who weighed nearly 400 pounds and who has lost almost 100 pounds also cannot believe how easy it has been to stay on the Race to Maintenance and how it has changed his life. Whether you have 20 or 200 pounds to lose this really works.

Personally, this was such a miracle for me. I was able to adhere to the Race to Maintenance requirements by following the Isagenix list of recommended foods, fats and complex carbohydrates. The great variety of recipes included in this book kept me within the healthy 600-calorie range for meals. I was able to lose a total of 30 pounds by doing 11-day cleanses and following them up with the Race to Maintenance program. That changed my life forever. I would never look back nor do I ever want to go back to where I was!

Nutritional Cleansing Coaches

The cleanse schedule and free coaching services offered through this program were equally as important to my success as the constant flow of nutrients. With encouragement and education, I was able to attain better results in both weight loss and overall health.

Anyone who enrolls in the program will be assigned a personal cleansing coach without charge. For me, the coaches were able to take out all the guesswork about how to properly utilize this nutritional technology. They developed and sent me daily schedules and assisted with any concerns or cleansing symptoms that occurred during my first few days of starting the program.

Although this is not a "one size fits all" program, everyone starts out very similarly to help fluidly integrate these nutrients into their lives. For people with any health struggles, the coaches can modify the program accordingly to make it a better fit for the individual.

Sustaining the Cleansing Lifestyle

People ask me all the time, "Do I have to do this for the rest of my life?" My answer is always the same. It starts with a question and that question is, "Why wouldn't you want to cleanse every day?" Toxins don't go on vacation once you stop the program.

An important reason you should continue drinking these whey protein shakes is that our bodies do not store proteins. Our bodies store fats and carbohydrates, but not protein. Plus, chicken, fish, soy and many other forms of protein just do not have the levels of ingredients our bodies need, such as the amino acids and the added ionic trace minerals.

Also (other than mother's breast milk), these whey protein shakes are simply unsurpassed as a source of protein to reduce the risk of sarcopenia (loss of muscle mass) and to supply your body with the nutrients that allow the body to continuing cleansing. The scientists certainly agree that un-denatured whey protein on its own is necessary for optimal health. With the addition of trace minerals and enzymes, IsaLean Shakes include ingredients that are essential to the human body. It's no wonder so many people call them "super shakes."

Now you can probably see why just consuming an IsaLean Shake each morning could give you so many advantages really over any other food you can possibly consume. It has so many benefits backed up by science that the real question you should ask yourself is "Why wouldn't I have an IsaLean Shake every morning for breakfast?" For me, it comes down to one simple concept: I cannot find a better food to put into my body each morning.

Super Shakes at a Glance

In addition to containing superior protein, these shakes are unique for many
reasons. Each "Super Shake" contains:

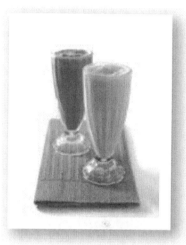

- 24 grams of New Zealand whey
protein and milk protein from
cows that are not injected with
antibiotics or growth hormones.
- Non-denatured protein processed
using low-temperature, high-fil-
tration pasteurization, as opposed
to high-heat pasteurization typically used in North America
that greatly reduces the amino acids available to the human
body.
- Protein from cows in New Zealand that are fed grass not corn.
- Eight grams of fiber, primarily from flax seed and prebiotic fiber, called isomaltooligosaccharides. Not all fiber is the same,
and this prebiotic fiber in particular is so important to our
bodies because it feeds healthy flora (good bacteria) in our
digestive tract. This is beneficial to our overall health.
- Whey protein and milk protein with a similar ratio that is
found in mother's breast milk, which is 60% whey protein and
40% milk protein.
- No artificial flavorings.
- No artificial sweeteners. Stevia is used as the sweetener (stevia contains no sugar and is naturally derived from the stevia

plant). As a result, these shakes taste great yet they have a very low glycemic index.

- High content of good fats, including olive oil, sunflower oil and coconut oil.
- No soy or soy-derived ingredients.
- No genetically modified (GMO) ingredients.
- Extremely low lactose combined with lactase, which is an enzyme that aids in the digestion of lactose.
- Protease, an enzyme that helps break down protein into particles called peptides that make the protein much easier to absorb.
- Gluten and wheat free.
- Canisters that the shakes are contained in are environmentally friendly because an ingredient has been added that completely breaks down the plastic, so there is no problem in landfills. These shakes are also available in foil packets as well.
- 70 alfalfa trace ionic minerals.
- Only 240 calories, yet it is a complete meal replacement. The great thing is that you feel really satisfied because of the massive amount of nutrients contained within each shake. Remember, the key to satisfying our hunger is nutritional density, not how many calories we eat.

If you can find a more nutritious or better food on this planet please let me know, so I can take it!

Maintenance and Plateaus

How do I sustain my results on a daily basis?

Every day, some level of cleansing is recommended for maintaining weight and, most importantly, optimal health. I've accomplished this by consuming two ounces of the Cleanse for Life® drink each morning, along with an IsaLean Shake. This way I the levels of necessary nutrients, vitamins and trace-minerals needed to maintain my fat-burning processes. I drink another two ounces of Cleanse for Life® before going to sleep, which continuously cleanses my body of everyday toxins and impurities. I also put my body through a two-day deep cleanse once every two months to rid it of those deeply embedded impurities trapped in fat cells.

Though it is important to continue to select from the list of recommended foods after completing the cleanse, it does not mean that "guilty pleasure" foods, such as pizza, ice cream or alcohol, cannot be enjoyed in a cleansing lifestyle—as long as they are consumed in moderation.

After completing the program, if you begin to experience food cravings again, or become fatigued, overwhelmed or depressed, this could be a warning sign that the body has gone back into sugar-burning mode. Sugar-burning mode is good for a very short period of time, such as when you are running a 100-yard dash. But the body was meant to burn fat for long-term energy. In sugar-burning mode you will constantly seek out sugars and carbs to replace the sugar that is rapidly used up. Fat burning produces much higher energy and much more long-term energy. The sooner you can get into and maintain fat burning, the more energy you will have and the better you will feel. You can combat sugar burning by immediately completing just one cleansing cycle to return your body to fat-burning mode.

As is the case with traditional diets, it is possible to hit a plateau. These plateau periods may indicate that the body has stopped burning fat—or that you have reintroduced simple carbohydrates, refined sugars or artificial sweeteners into your diet. This causes the body to enter starvation mode from the overconsumption of empty calories. Otherwise, the body may have achieved a state of equilibrium, and will retain fluid for a period of time until a new equilibrium point is set, at which time your body should dump the excess fluid. The key during any of these plateau periods is to not get discouraged, and to continue to self-motivate with the prospect of enhanced energy and full-rounded wellness in mind.

Once you are familiar with what to expect on each day of any cleansing program, you can introduce exercise into your daily routines. However, it is not recommended to start a cleanse and a new exercise program at the same time. When beginning this program, I was advised to walk a minimum of 30-60 minutes every day, preferably in the morning, to promote fat burning. Though I was told a 60-minute walk was ideal, if I could only walk for 15 minutes at a time. I walked twice a day for 15 minutes and then built myself up to 30 minutes. When I could, I also jumped on a trampoline for 30 minutes as a great form of daily exercise.

By combining exercise and these nutrient-rich foods, my body was able to function efficiently by burning fat for energy. I cannot stress enough that this was not merely a weight loss program for me; weight loss was a side benefit of my newfound cleansing lifestyle.

Adhering to the recommended regiment and consistently ingesting the rare combination of ingredients allowed my body to cleanse itself naturally so I could accomplish long-term optimal health and wellness, extend my longevity and maximize my personal potential.

The recommendations set forth in this program to achieve a cleansing lifestyle recognize toxicity as the cause for systemic problems throughout the body, and deal with the body as a whole to truly solve them. Although single-point solutions are helpful in specific applications, specific-point nutrients cannot deal with the systemic needs to maintain overall wellness of the body.

History has proven that new solutions are needed to update belief systems and eliminate the common misconceptions about nutritional science. To thrive on this toxic planet, we must continue to educate ourselves on the potentially harmful effects of our surroundings and vow to make changes in our daily lifestyles. Nutritional cleansing is a step toward reducing each of our own "toxic burdens" and ultimately sets us on the path toward long-term health.

Clinical Study

There have been thousands people who have had life-changing experiences using Isagenix products, but how does the Isagenix system quantitatively compare to a well-established heart-healthy diet? In September 2012, results of an independent, third-party clinical study[3] performed at the University of Illinois at Chicago (UIC) showed that people following the Isagenix system had superior results in many areas. The 10-week study evaluated the effects of two dietary plans—the Isagenix plan and a conventional "heart healthy" plan—in combination with intermittent fasting or cleanse days. The study measured body weight, body composition, cardiovascular risk factors and oxidative stress markers in 54 obese women with a body mass index above 35. Compared to the "heart healthy" group, the Isagenix subjects had the following results:

- 56% greater reduction in average weight loss
- 47% greater reduction in average body fat loss
- Twice as much visceral fat loss
- 35% greater reduction of oxidative stress
- Greater adherence in subjects
- Easier and more convenient

According to Isagenix Chief Science Officer Suk Cho, Ph.D., "When you see successful weight and visceral fat loss, the scientific literature suggests you should see a reduction in cardiovascular risk factors. This well designed clinical trial further supports the impact someone can have on his or her life by controlling calorie intake and using Isagenix."

---

3 For more details about this study and other health information see http://www.isagenixhealth.net/.

Conclusion

Once in a great while, something so extraordinary is discovered that it changes your life if you take advantage of it.

The toxic world we live in has been anxiously waiting for this life-changing discovery to be made.

This book has revealed this amazing discovery to you for the first time and made you aware of what is possible to live an extraordinary and healthier life.

Many of the scientists I have worked with are terrified at what is coming at us if we continue to do what we have been doing. We cannot expect different results. That is the definition of insanity.

How will we cope with three babies born every day who will develop diabetes in their lifetime? There will not be enough insulin.

How will we cope with projections that say in 30 years 100% of America will be overweight?

Can we afford to do nothing?

Can you afford to continue to do what you have been doing?

Even if you are a purist who does not drink or smoke and only eats organic and exercises regularly, these things are no longer enough if you are interested in living as long as you can and as healthy as you can.

The number of people who will become sick in the very near future will overwhelm the ability of drugs, health professionals, hospitals and drugs to deal with this oncoming Tsunami of obesity and health-related problems. We are a "sick-care" world already, and it is getting worse at an alarming rate. By the year 2112 it is estimated that nearly one million people will die of heart disease.

Some experts estimate that we now consume more than two trillion prescription drugs per year in North America. That represents nearly 50% of all the prescription drugs on earth. This is just today—not what is estimated will be required in the future.

In addition, our water, air and food are becoming more and more hostile to our very existence. We build mountains of food that lasts a long time on the shelf but does very little to sustain us minute-by-minute, hour-by-hour, day-by-day and month-by-month. As a result, each year we lose a little bit more of our ability to maximize our human potential no matter what our age.

We have learned very well to live this less-than-healthy lifestyle by tolerating being overweight, devoid of energy and loaded with stress and brain fog, as if this is the way it has to be. How bad does it have to get before you do something better for your body?

This book offers great hope and a real solution to a fate that may come your way if you do what you are currently doing and ignore the overwhelming evidence that a drastic new approach is needed. You are not alone. Instead of joining the legions of the sick you can now become one of the healthy who are fit, trim and full of energy. Maximize your full human potential and, most importantly, live healthier longer.

The cleanse is not a cure for anything. If the body is given dense nutrition it is capable of amazing things. I see this every day of my life. If we give the body the proper fuel, it simply functions better in all respects. As I said earlier, eat a low-quality form of protein and it takes your body several months to recover from the effects. There are simple things you can do that I've pointed out in this book. It is not a pipe dream or some broken promise; rather it is the reality of a cleansing lifestyle—and it attainable once you make a choice to do it.

I realize that most of you are as skeptical as I was. That skepticism is only natural given the choices we have all made. Like many of you, I had been disappointed over and over again with the next great breakthrough ("hope dope") in diet, health and nutrition, only to discover that it was too good to be true. And, yet when the next one came along I eagerly tried it, thinking this might be the one. Does that sound familiar?

So skepticism is an understandable reaction.

After many of these disappointing experiences, though, I have found that the Isagenix system is a major breakthrough in nutritional science. It is "the one." It is the real deal as they say. Never before, have so many people had consistent long-term, life-changing-results day after day, month after month, year after year. This is the first real long-term solution that can lead to a long-term healthy life.

Those who need to lose weight normally say "my scale must be broken" when they see dramatic weight loss.

Those who do the cleanse because they like the idea of giving their cells an "oil change" often say "I really did not believe it was possible to feel this good. I have more energy than I ever have had I just feel wonderful."

Athletes are amazed at the improvement in their lean muscle mass, drastic improvement in their athletic performance and their quick recovery time after working out.

This cleansing technology is not too good to be true; it is better than that. There are more than a million people who have done it safely with amazing results. And, it is for everyone, whether you are an athlete, healthy, overweight or not.

I invite you to just give us 11 days[4] and you can change your life. Your best years can truly be ahead of you if you are willing to adopt a cleansing life style now.

We realize you may still have questions before getting started, based on your own individual goals ,or maybe you just need more information. Our nutritional cleansing coaches are available to answer any and all of your questions, and if you do decide to join us they will coach you through the cleanse for free.

People ask me all the time, "Do I have to do this forever?" I just smile and say, "When you think the toxins are going on vacation and when the toxins do then you can stop."

If you can find a better food to put into your body each day please tell me and I will eat it!

---

4 This is the Isagenix 9-Day Cleanse and 2-Day Pre-Cleanse.

Your real desire to do the cleanse is simple: to live healthier for as long as you can. I don't know a single human being on this planet who is not interested in that.

I leave you to decide. As the famous scholar Hillel once said, "If I am not for myself, who will be for me?"

Results

Real people have seen real results with Isagenix. I know because it happened to me. My success is the reason I to believe that this nutritional cleansing technology was going to change my life—and it did.

Is it time for you to change your life now?

For more information, please feel free to contact us at: whydietsare-failingus.com or by calling us at 800-931-7810.

Bibliography

Acheson, K. et al. (2011). Protein choices targeting thermogenesis and metabolism. *The American Journal of Clinical Nutrition*, Vol. 93 No. 3 pp. 525-534.

Baillie-Hamilton, P. (2005). *Toxic Overload.* New York: Avery.

Beach, R. (1936). *Modern Miracle Men.* Washington, D.C.: U.S. Government Printing Office.

Campbell, W. et al. (2001). The recommended dietary allowance for protein may not be adequate for older people to maintain skeletal muscle. *Journal of Gerontology: Biological Sciences*, Vol. 56, Issue 6; pp. M373-M380.

Colgan, M. (2001). *The New Power Program: Protocols for Maximum Strength.* Apple Publishing Co.

Dangin, M. et al. (2001). The digestion rate of protein is an independent regulating factor of postprandial protein retention. *Am J Physiol Endocrinol Metab.*, Feb;280(2):E340-8.

Edwardes, C. (2003, September 14). Mr Banting's Old Diet Revolution. *The Telegraph.* London.

Encyclopædia Britannica. (2012). Retrieved July 30, 2012, from http://www.britannica.com/EBchecked/topic/90141/calorie

Enig, M. (1995). *Trans Fatty Acids in the Food Supply: A Comprehensive Report Covering 60 Years of Research.* Silver Spring, MD: Enig Associates, Inc.

Enig, M. (2000). *Know Your Fats : The Complete Primer for Understanding the Nutrition of Fats, Oils and Cholesterol.* Silver Spring, MD: Bethesda Press.

Enig, M.; Fallon, S. (1999). *Nourishing Traditions.* Washington, D.C.: New Trends Publishing.

Environmental Working Group. (2005, July 14). Study Finds Industrial Pollution Begins in the Womb. *News Release.* Washington, D.C.

EPA, U. (1990). *The National Human Adipose Tissue Survey.*

Fallon, S. (1996). Tripping Lightly Down the Prostaglandin Pathways. *Price-Pottenger Nutrition Foundation Health Journal,* 20:3:5-8.

Fallon, S. (2001). *Nourishing Traditions.* Washington, D.C.: New Trends Publishing.

Felton, C. et al. (1994). Dietary polyunsaturated fatty acids and compositions of human aortic plaque. *Lancet,* 344:1195-1196.

Finkelstein, E. (2012). Obesity and Severe Obesity Forecasts through 2030. *American Journal of Preventive Medicine,* Vol. 42, Issue 6, Pages 563-570.

Foxcroft, L. (2011). *Calories & Corsets: A History of Dieting Over 2000 Years.* London: Profile Books.

Gruber, B. (2002, May 25). *The History of Diets and Dieting.* Retrieved from CarbSmart: http://www.carbsmart.com/historydiets.html

Grun, F., & Blumberg, B. (2006). Environmental Obesogens: Organotins and Endocrine Disruption via Nuclear Receptor Signaling. *Endocrinology,* Vol. 147 No. 6 s50-s55.

Harper, D. (2012). Doctor of Osteopathy, Isagenix Scientific Advisory Board Chair.

Holtcamp, W. (2012). Obesogens: An Environmental Link to Obesity. *Environmental Health Perspective,* 120:a62-a68.

Houlihan, J., Kropp, T., Wiles, R., Gray, S., & Campbell, C. (2005). *Body Burden: The Pollution in Newborns.* Environmental Working Group.

Hyman, M. (2009). *The Ultra Mind Solution.* New York: Scribner.

Karnani, M. et al. (2011). Activation of Central Orexin/Hypocretin Neurons by Dietary Amino Acids. *Neuron,* 72: 616-629.

Kim,J; Li, Y; Watkins, B. (2011). Endocannabinoid signaling and energy metabolism: a target for dietary intervention. *Nutrition,* June 27 (6):624-32.

Lassek, W.; Gaulin, S. (2012). *Why Women Need Fat.* New York: Hudson Street Press.

Lasserre, M. et al. (1985). Effects of different dietary intake of essential fatty acids on C20:3 omega 6 and C20:4 omega 6 serum levels in human adults. *Lipids*, Apr;20(4):227-33.

Mann, T. et al. (2007, April). Medicare's Search for Effective Obesity Treatments: Diets Are Not the Answer. *American Psychologist*, pp. Vol. 62, No. 3, 220–233.

Miller, D. (2011). Retrieved from www.lewrockwell.com: http://www.lewrockwell.com/miller/miller38.1.html

National Institutes of Health. (2009, March 16). Study Helps Unravel Mysteries of Brain's Endocannabinoid System. U.S. Department of Health and Human Services.

Ogden, C.; Carroll, M. (2010). *Prevalence of Overweight, Obesity, and Extreme Obesity Among Adults: United States, Trends 1960–1962 Through 2007–2008.* Centers for Disease Control and Prevention.

Pennings, B. et al. (2011, May). Whey protein stimulates postprandial muscle protein accretion more effectively than do casein and casein hydrolysate in older men. *The American Journal of Clinical Nutrition*, pp. 93(5):997-1005.

Perrine, S. (2010). *The New American Diet.* Rodale Inc.

Peters, L. H. (1918). *Diet and Health: With Key to The Calories.* Chicago: The Reilly & Lee Co.

Pimentel, D. L. (1986). *Pesticides: Amounts Applied and Amounts Reaching Pests.* American Institute of Biological Sciences.

Pinckney, E. et al. (1973). *The Cholesterol Controversy*. Los Angeles: Sherbourne Press.

Pollan, M. (2006). *The Omnivore's Dilemma*. New York: The Penguin Press.

Schauss, M. (2008). *Achieving Victory Over a Toxic World*. Bloomington, IN: AuthorHouse.

Stitt, P. (1982). *Beating the Food Giants*. Natural Press.

STOP Obesity Alliance Research Team. (2010). *Improving Obesity Management in*. Washington, D.C.: The George Washington University School of Public Health and Health Services.

The Endocrine Society. (2009). *Endocrine-Disrupting Chemicals*. Chevy Chase, MD.

USDA. (2011). *Sugar and Sweeteners Outlook, No. (SSSM-273)*. Washington, D.C.: U.S. Department of Agriculture.

Valero-Garrido, D. et al. (1990). Influence of Dietary Fat on the Lipid Composition of Perirenal Adipose Tissue in Rats. *Annals of Nutrition and Metabolism*, 34:327-332.

vom Saal, F. et al. (2012). The estrogenic endocrine disrupting chemical bisphenol A (BPA) and obesity. *Molecular and Cellular Endocrinology*, 354: 74-84.

Weinberg, B., & Bealer, B. (2001). *The World of Caffeine: The Science and Culture of the World's Most Popular Drug*. New York: Routledge.

Wilkinson, A. (1995, June 5). Oh, What A Tangled Web. *The New Yorker*, p. 34.

Wilson, L. (2011). *Selenium: A Critical Mineral for Health and Healing.* Prescott, AZ: Center for Development.

Appendix I _____

18 Reasons to Try This Life Changing Cleansing Technology

1. **Liver Support...** the liver is the main detoxifying organ of the body. It takes fat-soluble toxins so that they can be excreted in the urine. This is made easier with the amino acids in Isagenix products.

2. **Antioxidant Protection...** free radicals damage cells. Antioxidants are substances that fight free radicals.

3. **Aids in the Loss of Weight...** it's proven that weight loss decreases the chances of diabetes, cancer and heart disease thus increasing your life expectancy.

4. **Enhanced Mental Abilities...** a recent study showed that mental abilities improve with weight loss. Many Isagenix users report weight loss as a benefit.

5. **Increased Energy...** do you want to feel better and accomplish more? Isagenix isn't an "energy drink," but rather delivers a level of nutrition that will help you get more done each day without feeling like you have been overworked.

6. **Immune Support...** cleansing the body of impurities while replenishing it with vital nutrients can improve immune function and lessen immunity threats within the body.

7. **Better Cellular Function...** our cells need essential nutrients and compounds to be healthy and communicate. Nutritional cleansing delivers such nutrients and creates an environment where cells can effectively communicate and perform.

8. **Premature-Aging Protection...** nutrient deficiencies, impurities and toxins can damage our cells and organs and lead to premature aging. Nutritional cleansing slows the onslaught of the toxic world and creates a shield of protection for increased energy and a sense of overall rejuvenation.

9. **Better Digestion...** Isagenix delivers enzymes and other vital nutrients for the digestive tract. The digestive system is replenished with good bacteria and enzymes to help with the breakdown and absorption of food.

10. **Enhanced Nutrition...** the best way to take control of your health is through improved nutrition. One of the few things in life that you can control is: you get to decide what goes into your body - and what goes into your body determines what type of body you will have. Isagenix products are a terrific nutrition source.

11. **Weight Control...** it's no secret that obesity is a huge problem in today's society. Many degenerative diseases are associated with obesity, either as the cause or a complicating

factor. Cleansing may help support the loss of excess fat and water and increase muscle mass.

12. **Fights Obesity...** obesity is on the rise and has been rising since 1985 when the CDC (Center for Disease Control and Prevention) started to monitor obesity. It is now estimated that almost 26% of the adult population is obese or morbidly obese. Nutritional cleansing as part of a healthy lifestyle can reduce the likelihood of obesity.

13. **Adaptogenic Support...** some of the Isagenix products contain adaptogens, which have been used by Olympic athletes for years. Adaptogens are agents (usually botanicals) that help the body "adapt" to physical and mental stress.

14. **Less Cravings...** as you cleanse it's very common to have cravings for unhealthy foods go away. These cravings are replaced with a sense of well-being and satiety.

15. **An "Aura" of Wellness...** want to look good and have that air of good health and energy? It's almost impossible to do this if you're not eating nutritionally dense foods like those from Isagenix.

16. **Youthful Skin...** skin cannot be healthy without the proper nutrition from the inside. This also applies for impurities in the body. Cleansing and replenishing your body with vital nutrients can lead to smooth, youthful-looking skin.

17. **Rejuvenation with Trace Minerals...** Isagenix products contain ionic minerals, which are the key to a healthy body. Cells cannot function properly without them. Ionic minerals

are easily absorbed and, once in the body, speed up innumerable cellular reactions.

18. **Gastrointestinal Support...** replacing poor-quality, low-fiber foods with high-quality, nutritionally dense foods can improve digestion and enhance gastrointestinal function.

Appendix II

Sample Chart: 9-Day Cleanse and 2-Day Pre-Cleanse

Your Bridge to a Cleansing LifeStyle
Isagenix 9-Day Cleanse For Life Program

Pre-Cleanse · 2 Days

7:00am	*Breakfast* 2 scoops of IsaLean Shake mixed with 8oz of water & ice / Drink 8 to 16oz of water 1 Natural Accelerator Capsule
9:00am	Small handful of nuts (unsalted, dry roasted: almonds, walnuts, pine nuts or Brazil nuts) / Drink 8 to 16oz of water
10:30am	Small handful of nuts (unsalted, dry roasted: almonds, walnuts, pine nuts or Brazil nuts) / Drink 8 to 16oz of water
12:30pm	*Lunch* Enjoy one regular meal of approximately 400-600 calories. / Drink 8 to 16oz water 1 Natural Accelerator Capsule
2:00pm	Small handful of nuts (unsalted, dry roasted: almonds, walnuts, pine nuts or Brazil nuts) / Drink 8 to 16oz of water
3:30pm	Small handful of nuts (unsalted, dry roasted: almonds, walnuts, pine nuts or Brazil nuts) / Drink 8 to 16oz of water
5:00pm	*Dinner* 2 scoops of IsaLean Shake mixed with 8oz of water & ice / Drink 8 to 16oz of water
6:30pm	Small handful of nuts (unsalted, dry roasted: almonds, walnuts, pine nuts or Brazil nuts) / Drink 8 to 16oz of water
8:30pm	Small handful of nuts (unsalted, dry roasted: almonds, walnuts, pine nuts or Brazil nuts) / Drink 8 to 16oz of water

Key Points:
- For BEST results, eat your meal at lunch.
- Remember your nuts. Your Isagenix Snacks will begin on Day 1 (see next page).
- Stay active - light walking or bouncing is great to stimulate your lymphatic system.
- Drink plenty of water ... for cleansing and also for the importance to our overall health and wellness. Drink no more than half of your body weight in oz of water.

Call your support coach if you are uncomfortable at any time. Your coach can help you. There are many solutions and options with the Isagenix System.

Coach_____ Phone#_____

Day 1 & 2 · Cleanse

7:00am	*Breakfast* 4oz Cleanse For Life Drink mixed with 8oz of cold water / Drink 8 to 16oz of water 1 Natural Accelerator Capsule
9:00am	Isagenix Snack and 2 almonds / Drink 8 to 16oz of water
10:30am	Isagenix Snack / Drink 8 to 16oz of water
12:30pm	*Lunch* 4oz Cleanse For Life Drink mixed with 8oz of cold water / Drink 8 to 16oz of water 1 Natural Accelerator Capsule
2:00pm	Isagenix Snack and 2 almonds / Drink 8 to 16oz of water
3:30pm	Isagenix Snack / Drink 8 to 16oz of water
5:00pm	*Dinner* 4oz Cleanse For Life Drink mixed with 8oz of cold water / Drink 8 to 16oz of water
6:30pm	Isagenix Snack and 2 almonds / Drink 8 to 16oz of water
8:00pm	*Evening* 4oz Cleanse For Life Drink mixed with 8oz of cold water
9:30pm	Isagenix Snack and 2 almonds / Drink 8 to 16oz of water

Key Points:
- Do not let more than 2 hours pass without a meal or snack. Isagenix Snacks stabilize blood sugar levels and the Natural Accelerator capsule supports a healthy metabolism.
- NO solid food on Cleanse days.
- Remember your water! If you start to get a headache it is usually an indicator of not consuming enough water – drink 8-16 oz of water immediately.
- If you find your cleanse day a bit challenging, you may eat a small handful of nuts, or a piece of celery.
- Rest and honor your body during this time – your body is working really hard.
- Exercise should be light so that you increase circulation without expending too many calories. Take a walk or do a light yoga workout.
- Ask your Coach about the Race to Maintenance Program on Day 3.

Replenish | Day 3-7

7:00am   *Breakfast* 2 scoops of IsaLean Shake mixed with 8oz of water & ice / Drink 8 to 16oz of water
       1 Natural Accelerator Capsule

9:00am   Isagenix Snack and 2 almonds / Drink 8 to 16oz of water

10:30am   Isagenix Snack and 2 almonds / Drink 8 to 16oz of water

12:30pm   *Lunch* Enjoy one regular meal of approximately 400-600 calories. / Drink 8 to 16oz of water
       1 Natural Accelerator Capsule

2:00pm   Isagenix Snack and 2 almonds / Drink 8 to 16oz of water

3:30pm   Isagenix Snack and 2 almonds / Drink 8 to 16oz of water

5:00pm   *Dinner* 2 scoops of IsaLean Shake mixed with 8oz of water & ice / Drink 8 to 16oz of water

6:30pm   Isagenix Snack and 2 almonds / Drink 8 to 16oz of water

8:30pm   Isagenix Snack and 2 almonds / Drink 8 to 16oz of water

Key Points:
- For BEST results eat your meal at lunch. Meals may also be split into two smaller portion meals – your Isagenix Shake is the last meal of the day. Organic is best. Eat 4 to 6 oz of lean protein such as chicken, turkey, fish, seafood or grass fed beef; 3 to 4 cups of vegetables (i.e. romaine lettuce, cabbage, bell peppers, green beans, tomatoes, celery, cucumbers, artichoke hearts, bok choy, broccoli, cauliflower, avocados, eggplant...) - they may be eaten raw as a salad, or you may steam them until tender.
- Remember to eat your Isagenix Snacks.
- Stay active, light walking or bouncing is great to stimulate your lymphatic system. The lymphatic system carries the impurities from the cells into the blood stream then into the colon.
- Place your next order on Day 3 to allow for shipping time – you're feeling great now and you want to continue burning fat (not sugar) to look and feel your absolute best!

Day 8-9 | *Revitalize*

7:00am   *Breakfast* 4oz Cleanse For Life Drink mixed with 8oz of cold water / Drink 8 to 16oz of water
       1 Natural Accelerator Capsule

9:00am   Isagenix Snack and 2 almonds / Drink 8 to 16oz of water

10:30am   Isagenix Snack and 2 almonds / Drink 8 to 16oz of water

12:30pm   *Lunch* 4oz Cleanse For Life Drink mixed with 8oz of cold water / Drink 8 to 16oz of water
       1 Natural Accelerator Capsule

2:00pm   Isagenix Snack and 2 almonds / Drink 8 to 16oz of water

3:30pm   Isagenix Snack and 2 almonds / Drink 8 to 16oz of water

5:00pm   *Dinner* 4oz Cleanse For Life Drink mixed with 8oz of cold water / Drink 8 to 16oz of water

6:30pm   Isagenix Snack and 2 almonds / Drink 8 to 16oz of water

8:00pm   *Evening* 4oz Cleanse For Life Drink mixed with 8oz of cold water

9:30pm   Isagenix Snack and 2 almonds / Drink 8 to 16oz of water

- Continue taking your Natural Accelerator Capsules – you have a 30-day supply

Key Points:
- Blend the Cleanse for Life drink with water and ice to enjoy as a slushy!
- Relax, enjoy and be at peace. Curl up with a good book. Rent a good movie. Your body is working really hard on the inside – you've earned the time to relax!
- Talk with your Coach about the 30-Day Race to Maintenance options to continue to revitalize your health, as well as maintain optimum health and wellness.
- This is the beginning of the rest of your life! What you've experienced will keep getting better and better as you continue to use the products. Ask about our Autoship program to assist you in leading a cleansing lifestyle.

NOTE: Are people starting to ask you what you've been doing? Your coach can help you with what to say. It may surprise you that by simply sharing your story, you could earn your products for FREE!

Appendix III

Sample Chart: Race to Maintenance

Isagenix *Race to Maintenance*
(Follows the Isagenix 9-Day Program)

Shake/Meal/Meal/Shake — Day 10-14

7:00am	*Breakfast* 2 scoops of IsaLean Shake mixed with 8oz of water & ice / Drink 8 to 16oz of water 1 Natural Accelerator Capsule
9:00am	Isagenix Snack and 2 almonds* / Drink 8 to 16oz of water
10:30am	Isagenix Snack and 2 almonds* / Drink 8 to 16oz of water
12:30pm	*Lunch* Enjoy one regular meal of approximately 400-600 calories. / Drink 8 to 16oz of water 1 Natural Accelerator Capsule
2:00pm	Isagenix Snack and 2 almonds* / Drink 8 to 16oz of water
3:30pm	Isagenix Snack and 2 almonds* / Drink 8 to 16oz of water
6:00pm	*Dinner* Enjoy one regular meal of approximately 400-600 calories. / Drink 8 to 16oz of water
7:30pm	2 scoops of IsaLean Shake mixed with 8oz of water & ice / Drink 8 to 16oz of water
9:00pm	Isagenix Snack and 2 almonds* / Drink 8 to 16oz of water

Key Points:
- * Enjoy up to 6 Isagenix Snacks per day. Take as needed.
- Drink plenty of water throughout the day. The maximum you want to drink is one-half of your body weight in ounces.
- Stay active - light walking or bouncing is great to stimulate your lymphatic system and carry the impurities from your body. Call your support coach if you are uncomfortable at any time or have questions. Your coach can help you. There are many solutions and options with the Isagenix System.

Coach_____ Phone#_____

Day 15-16 — *Cleanse*

7:00am	*Breakfast* 4oz Cleanse For Life Drink mixed with 8oz of cold water / Drink 8 to 16oz of water 1 Natural Accelerator Capsule
9:00am	Isagenix Snack and 2 almonds / Drink 8 to 16oz of water
10:30am	Isagenix Snack / Drink 8 to 16oz of water
12:30pm	*Lunch* 4oz Cleanse For Life Drink mixed with 8oz of cold water / Drink 8 to 16oz of water 1 Natural Accelerator Capsule
2:00pm	Isagenix Snack and 2 almonds / Drink 8 to 16oz of water
3:30pm	Isagenix Snack / Drink 8 to 16oz of water
5:00pm	*Dinner* 4oz Cleanse For Life Drink mixed with 8oz of cold water / Drink 8 to 16oz of water
6:30pm	Isagenix Snack and 2 almonds / Drink 8 to 16oz of water
8:00pm	*Evening* 4oz Cleanse For Life Drink mixed with 8oz of cold water
9:30pm	Isagenix Snack and 2 almonds / Drink 8 to 16oz of water

Key Points:
- Do not let more than 2 hours pass without a meal or snack.
- Remember your water! If you start to get a headache it is usually an indicator of not consuming enough water - drink 8-16 oz of water immediately.
- If you are having a hard time on your cleanse days, you may want to supplement with a small handful of nuts, or a piece of celery.
- Rest and honor your body during this time.
- Exercise should be light so that you increase circulation without expending too many calories. Take a walk or do a light yoga workout.

Shake/<u>Meal</u>/<u>Meal</u>/Shake

Day 17-21

7:00am	*Breakfast* 2 scoops of IsaLean Shake mixed with 8oz of water & Ice / Drink 8 to 16oz of water 1 Natural Accelerator Capsule
9:00am	Isagenix Snack and 2 almonds* / Drink 8 to 16oz of water
10:30am	Isagenix Snack and 2 almonds* / Drink 8 to 16oz of water
12:30pm	*Lunch* Enjoy one regular meal of approximately 400-600 calories. / Drink 8 to 16oz of water 1 Natural Accelerator Capsule
2:00pm	Isagenix Snack and 2 almonds* / Drink 8 to 16oz of water
3:30pm	Isagenix Snack and 2 almonds* / Drink 8 to 16oz of water
6:00pm	*Dinner* Enjoy one regular meal of approximately 400-600 calories. / Drink 8 to 16oz of water
7:30pm	2 scoops of IsaLean Shake mixed with 8oz of water & Ice / Drink 8 to 16oz of water
9:00pm	Isagenix Snack and 2 almonds* / Drink 8 to 16oz of water

Key Points:
- For BEST results eat organic. Eat 4 to 6 oz of lean protein such as chicken, turkey, fish, seafood or grass fed beef; 3 to 4 cups of vegetables (i.e. romaine lettuce, cabbage, bell peppers, green beans, tomatoes, celery, cucumbers, artichoke hearts, bok choy, broccoli, cauliflower, avocados, eggplant...) - they may be eaten raw as a salad, or you may steam them until tender.
- *Enjoy up to 6 Isagenix Snacks per day. Take as needed.
- Drink plenty of water throughout the day. The maximum water you want to drink is one-half of your body weight in ounces.
- Stay active - light walking or bouncing is great.

Day 22-23

Cleanse

7:00am	*Breakfast* 4oz Cleanse For Life Drink mixed with 8oz of cold water / Drink 8 to 16oz of water 1 Natural Accelerator Capsule
9:00am	Isagenix Snack and 2 almonds / Drink 8 to 16oz of water
10:30am	Isagenix Snack / Drink 8 to 16oz of water
12:30pm	*Lunch* 4oz Cleanse For Life Drink mixed with 8oz of cold water / Drink 8 to 16oz of water 1 Natural Accelerator Capsule
2:00pm	Isagenix Snack and 2 almonds / Drink 8 to 16oz of water
3:30pm	Isagenix Snack / Drink 8 to 16oz of water
5:00pm	*Dinner* 4oz Cleanse For Life Drink mixed with 8oz of cold water / Drink 8 to 16oz of water
6:30pm	Isagenix Snack and 2 almonds / Drink 8 to 16oz of water
8:00pm	*Evening* 4oz Cleanse For Life Drink mixed with 8oz of cold water
9:30pm	Isagenix Snack and 2 almonds / Drink 8 to 16oz of water

Key Points:
- Finish strong, you're doing great!
- Place your next order 30 days from your last order to allow for shipping time - you're feeling great now and do not want to run out. Call your coach now to schedule a convenient time within the next week to discuss the program that is best suited for you moving forward. Remember, your coach can explain the various programs, as well as talk with you about other products and programs that may help you with your health and financial goals!
- Ask about our Autoship benefits.

NOTE: Are people starting to ask you what you've been doing? Your coach can help you with what to say. It may surprise you that by simply sharing your story, you could earn your products for FREE!

Shake/*Meal*/*Meal*/Shake — Day 24-28

7:00am *Breakfast* 2 scoops of IsaLean Shake mixed with 8oz of water & ice / Drink 8 to 16oz of water
1 Natural Accelerator Capsule

9:00am Isagenix Snack and 2 almonds* / Drink 8 to 16oz of water

10:30am Isagenix Snack and 2 almonds* / Drink 8 to 16oz of water

12:30pm *Lunch* Enjoy one regular meal of approximately 400-600 calories. / Drink 8 to 16oz of water
1 Natural Accelerator Capsule

2:00pm Isagenix Snack and 2 almonds* / Drink 8 to 16oz of water

3:30pm Isagenix Snack and 2 almonds* / Drink 8 to 16oz of water

6:00pm *Dinner* Enjoy one regular meal of approximately 400-600 calories. / Drink 8 to 16oz of water

7:30pm 2 scoops of IsaLean Shake mixed with 8oz of water & ice / Drink 8 to 16oz of water

9:00pm Isagenix Snack and 2 almonds* / Drink 8 to 16oz of water

Key Points:
- For BEST results eat organic. Eat 4 to 6 oz of lean protein such as chicken, turkey, fish, seafood or grass fed beef; 3 to 4 cups of vegetables (i.e. romaine lettuce, cabbage, bell peppers, green beans, tomatoes, celery, cucumbers, artichoke hearts, bok choy, broccoli, cauliflower, avocados, eggplant...) - they may be eaten raw as a salad, or you may steam them until tender.
- *Enjoy up to 6 Isagenix Snacks per day. Take as needed.
- Drink plenty of water throughout the day. The maximum water you want to drink is one-half of your body weight in ounces.
- Stay active - light walking or bouncing is great.
- 1-2 IsaDelight™ mid-morning and mid-afternoon on an empty stomach (must be taken either 15 minutes prior to your cleanse drink, snacks and nuts, or 1 ½ hours after cleanse, snacks and nuts) can replace an Isagenix Snack twice a day.

Day 29-30 — *Cleanse*

7:00am *Breakfast* 4oz Cleanse For Life Drink mixed with 8oz of cold water / Drink 8 to 16oz of water
1 Natural Accelerator Capsule

9:00am Isagenix Snack and 2 almonds / Drink 8 to 16oz of water

10:30am Isagenix Snack / Drink 8 to 16oz of water

12:30pm *Lunch* 4oz Cleanse For Life Drink mixed with 8oz of cold water / Drink 8 to 16oz of water
1 Natural Accelerator Capsule

2:00pm Isagenix Snack and 2 almonds / Drink 8 to 16oz of water

3:30pm Isagenix Snack / Drink 8 to 16oz of water

5:00pm *Dinner* 4oz Cleanse For Life Drink mixed with 8oz of cold water / Drink 8 to 16oz of water

6:30pm Isagenix Snack and 2 almonds / Drink 8 to 16oz of water

8:00pm *Evening* 4oz Cleanse For Life Drink mixed with 8oz of cold water

9:30pm Isagenix Snack and 2 almonds / Drink 8 to 16oz of water

Key Points:
- Finish strong, you're doing great!
- Call your coach now to schedule a convenient time within the next week to discuss the program that is best suited for you moving forward. Remember, your coach can explain the various programs, as well as talk with you about other products and programs that may help you with your health and financial goals!
- Ask about our Autoship benefits.

NOTE: Are people starting to ask you what you've been doing? Your coach can help you with what to say. It may surprise you that by simply sharing your story, you could earn your products for FREE!

Appendix IV _____

Recipes for Your Success

You are not alone and this is why we have put together some wonderful recipes to get you started.

These recipes have been carefully put together to give you plenty of choices. The following recipes and vegetarian alternatives are recommended as lunch options to be eaten during the program or as a delicious and healthy meal anytime. All the recipes include acceptable and suggested foods to integrate into your diet if you choose to partake in the Isagenix cleanse and begin your personal journey to full wellness. Enjoy!

Radical Red Potato Salad

1 cup red potato—cut into
   bite size pieces
1 cup chicken broth (low
   sodium, so you control
   the seasoning)
1 cup water
1 tsp. sea salt

1 tbsp. white wine vinegar
2 hard-boiled eggs
1 stalk celery
1 tbsp. parsley
¼ cup chopped red onion
½ cup steamed broccoli

Simmer potatoes in the above brine mixture of chicken broth, water, salt and vinegar for 15 minutes on medium low, and then boil on high for 2 minutes to reduce the liquid. Drain the potatoes reserving ⅛ cup of the liquid. Place potatoes in a serving bowl.

Dressing:

⅛ cup of reserved potato
   liquid
⅛ cup olive oil
1 tsp. white wine vinegar

1 tsp. Dijon mustard
⅛ cup of the cooked
   potatoes (optional)

Blend the above dressing mixture together (the addition of cooked potatoes thickens the dressing a bit). Pour the dressing over the potatoes in the bowl. Then add the chopped celery, parsley and red onion. Mix and toss. Season with salt and pepper. Serve at room temperature with steamed broccoli on the side.

Quinoa Pilaf with Swiss Chard, Toasted Pine Nuts

1 cup quinoa
2 cups vegetable or
   mushroom broth
3 tbsp. pine nuts
¼ cup sun dried tomatoes
1 tbsp. olive oil
2 cups uncooked Swiss
   chard

1 clove garlic, chopped
¼ cup garbanzo beans
   (chick peas)
½ tsp. paprika
½ pepper
¼ tsp. sea salt

In saucepan, put in 1 cup quinoa, 2 cups broth, salt, pepper, and paprika. Bring to a boil. Immediately turn down heat and let simmer for 10-15 min. While quinoa is cooking, heat ½ tbsp. olive oil on low heat in skillet and add pine nuts. Toast for 2 min, watching carefully not to overcook them. When nuts are lightly browned, add the other ½ tbsp. olive oil and garlic. Add Swiss chard and sauté for just a moment until wilted. Toss the nuts, Swiss chard, and sun-dried tomatoes into quinoa. Feel free to experiment with substitutions, as this can be a creative dish. The broth both flavors the quinoa nicely and also adds good minerals.

Fiesta Black Beans and Rice with Green Salad

½ cup dried black beans

2 strips kombu (seaweed)

½ cup uncooked brown rice

1 cup water

1 yellow onion

2 cups mixed greens

½ tsp. cumin

½ tsp. chili powder

1 clove garlic

Juice from 1 lime

½ tsp. sea salt

¼ cup fresh cilantro

1 small fresh tomato

The night before you wish to have this dish, soak the black beans in water. Drain the following day. Cook on low or in a crock pot with fresh water the next day with seaweed strips, yellow onion, and salt for a couple hours or until tender. In a saucepan, combine cooked brown rice, cumin, chili powder, garlic, and salt with 1 cup water. Bring to a boil, then immediately reduce heat and simmer for 10-15 minutes. Lay the mixed greens on a plate and pour the brown rice and black beans on top. Squeeze lime juice from over the top and garnish with cilantro and fresh tomato.

Harvest Roasted and Stuffed Butternut Squash

1 medium butternut squash, halved and seeded
1 clove garlic, minced
1 cup cooked barley (hulled or hulless)
½ tsp. sea salt
½ tsp. pepper
½ tsp. sage
½ tsp. rosemary
1 tsp. olive oil
½ thyme
1 carrot
½ cup mushrooms
2 tbsp. walnuts, chopped

Preheat oven to 400°. Place squash in foil and put into a baking dish with olive oil and bake until tender, approximately 50 minutes. Cook barley with sea salt (with a ratio of 2:1 water to barley) for about 45 minutes. In a skillet, sauté garlic, carrots, mushrooms with sage, rosemary, thyme, and pepper. Combine vegetable mixture with barley and stir in walnuts, mixing well. Divide barley and vegetable mixture between the two halves of the butternut squash.

Carrot coconut and Ginger Bisque and Baby Butter Lettuce Salad

Bisque:

2 tsp. coconut oil

1 medium onion, chopped

3 tbsp. finely chopped fresh
   ginger root

3 cups carrots, chopped

1 medium potato, peeled
   and chopped

8 cups vegetable stock

1 can coconut milk (13 oz.)

Fresh parsley or cilantro,
   chopped (optional)

Heat the coconut oil in a large pot. Add the onion and ginger and sauté just until the onion is translucent. Add the carrots, potato and vegetable stock. Bring to a boil, cover, reduce heat and boil gently until the vegetables are tender, about 30-45 minutes. Purée the soup in batches in a blender or food processor. Add salt to taste and gently swirl in coconut milk. Serve plain or garnished with chopped fresh parsley or cilantro.

Salad:

1 small head of baby butter
   lettuce

1 slice red onion

½ avocado

Toasted shaved almonds

½ fresh mango, sliced

Spicy citrus dressing:

Juice of 1 lemon

2 tbsp. chopped shallots

2 tbsp. white wine vinegar

¾ cup extra-virgin olive oil

Pinch of cayenne

2 pinches of both salt and
pepper

Wash and shred the butter lettuce. Top with sliced red onion, bite-sized avocado, toasted almond and fresh mango slices. Toss in the spicy citrus dressing. This salad accents the bisque by using mango to complement the coconut, and also adds the warmth of ginger and cayenne to support digestion.

Miso Soup with Ginger and Root Veggies

3 cups vegetable stock
1 tsp. miso paste
1 tbsp. dried wakame (or any seaweed, i.e. nori, kombu)
1 cup chopped kale
½ lb. shitake or portabella mushrooms

⅛ yellow onion, sliced
1 carrot peeled and chopped
1 celeriac root (celery root) peeled and chopped
1 tbsp. chopped ginger
2 cloves garlic, chopped
¼ cup uncooked quinoa

Pour stock into pot or large sauté pan. Add seaweed and simmer for 5 minutes. Add onion, carrot and other veggies. Sauté for 2 minutes. Add ginger, kale and shitake mushrooms and sauté for 3 minutes. Add garlic and uncooked quinoa and simmer for 15 minutes. Remove from heat and add miso paste that's been mixed with a little water or broth. Do not boil miso, it will kill the beneficial enzymes.

Golden Lentil and Sweet Potato Stew

½ cup dry yellow lentils
¾ cup chopped sweet
   potato
1 tbsp. ghee (clarified butter)
½ yellow onion
1 large carrot, chopped
1 clove garlic, minced
1 large celery stalk, chopped

¼ cup fresh parsley,
   chopped
½ tsp. sea salt
½ tsp. pepper
½ tsp. onion powder
½ tsp. garam masala
2 cups water
3 leaves of spinach chopped

Put 2 cups of water and lentils into small pot with chopped sweet potato and salt and bring to a boil. Immediately lower heat and let simmer 30 minutes. While lentils are cooking, sauté garlic, onion, carrot, and celery in olive oil. When lentils are cooked add vegetable mixture, pepper, onion powder, and garam masala. Simmer for another 15 minutes. Add spinach greens for just a minute. When cooking is complete stir in fresh parsley and salt to taste. This is a great recipe to use up extra veggies. It is easy to heat up and very filling.

Miso Sesame Roasted Tempeh and Cauliflower with Spinach

3–4 oz. tempeh
1 cup cauliflower
1 tbsp. miso paste
1 tbsp. rice wine vinegar
¼ cup water or vegetable broth

2 tbsp. sesame oil
1 tbsp. coconut oil
2–3 cups spinach, packed
Dash of Siracha (optional)
2 tsp. black sesame seeds

Cut the tempeh into triangles. In a small bowl, whisk together miso, rice wine vinegar, water or broth until the mixture is a thin paste. Thin it out with water or broth if necessary. Toss the tempeh and cauliflower in paste until gently coated. Sprinkle with black sesame seeds. Place in a baking dish in the oven on 350° for about 10–15 minutes.

In a skillet briefly sauté spinach in coconut oil until barely wilted. Finish with a dash of sesame oil, optional Siracha, and a sprinkle of sea salt. Serve the tempeh and cauliflower on a bed of spinach for a delicious and easy meal.

Spinach and Goat Cheese Frittata

1 garlic clove
1 zucchini
1 small shallot
2 eggs
1 ½ cups chopped spinach
1 tbsp. butter
1 small red bell pepper,
    chopped

½ tsp. sea salt
½ black pepper
½ cup chopped mushrooms
3 cherry tomatoes
½ tsp. red pepper flakes
    (optional)
¼ cup goat cheese

Preheat oven to 350°. Sauté garlic, onion, and pepper in butter. When almost cooked, add in zucchini, mushrooms, and spinach and cook until spinach is slightly wilted. In separate bowl, whisk together eggs, salt, pepper, and red pepper flakes. Add vegetables and stir in goat cheese crumbles, and chopped cherry tomatoes. Pour mixture into small cake pan that has been greased and bake for 30 minutes. Let frittata cool for about 5 minutes before serving.

Roasted Acorn Squash with Mushroom Gravy and Green Beans

1 small acorn squash
2 cups sliced mushrooms
  (shitake, portabella,
  chanterelle, oyster, etc.)
1–2 tsp. miso paste
2 cloves garlic
¼ cup onion
¼ tsp. umboshi plum
  vinegar

¼ cup nutritional yeast
  (available in health food
  stores)
sea salt to taste
½ to 1 cup water
⅛ cup olive oil
1 cup fresh green beans
2 tsp. slivered almonds

Cut and acorn squash in half and scoop out the seeds. Place the squash on a baking sheet and bake at 350° for about 30 minutes or until soft to the touch. In a skillet, sauté garlic and onion in olive oil until transparent and aromatic. Add mushrooms and let them cook down until soft, add water as needed. Add the water, nutritional yeast, vinegar and sea salt to taste. Simmer until well-cooked down. Remove from heat and add miso paste that has been blended with a little water. Steam the green beans until bright green and still a bit crunchy. Scoop out the insides of the squash and arrange green beans on top. Pour the mushroom mixture over squash and steamed green beans and top with slivered almonds. This is a delicious and nutritionally dense meal.

Roasted Fennel and Veggies in a Balsamic Glaze

½ onion, sliced in chunks
1 parsnip
½ cup chopped red, green and/or yellow bell peppers cut in large chunks
½ fennel root cut in chunks

3–4 of garlic cloves peeled (leave them whole or halve them)
1 ½ tbsp. olive oil
1 tbsp. balsamic vinegar
½ cup course corn meal
¼ tsp. sea salt (or to taste)

Roast Vegetables:

Place fennel and veggies in a large open baking dish and toss generously with olive oil and balsamic vinegar, salt and pepper to taste. Roast at 350° for about 30 minutes.

Polenta:

Bring 1 cup water or low-sodium chicken broth to a boil. Reduce to a simmer. Pour in corn meal steadily, stirring constantly. Cover and cook on low heat for 40–50 minutes, stirring every 10 minutes or so until polenta is thickened. It should come away from sides of the pan, and be able to support a spoon. Pour polenta onto a wooden cutting board to cool once it is solid, let stand for a few minutes. Serve with roasted vegetables.

Turnip Puff with Seared Rainbow Chard

Turnips are a delicious root vegetable that are super high in minerals, vitamin C and folic acid. Feel free to use green chard in place of rainbow chard.

1 small turnip, cubed
2 tbsp. ghee (clarified butter)
2 eggs, beaten
2 tsp. potato starch
1 tsp. maple syrup
1 tsp. baking powder
Pinch of sea salt or tamari

generous sprinkle of pepper
¼ cup dry bread crumbs
1 bundle of rainbow chard,
  de-stemmed and torn
  into bite size pieces
1 tsp. coconut oil

Cook the turnip in salted water until tender. Combine turnip, ghee and eggs. Mix dry ingredients together and add to the turnip mixture. Put into a greased casserole dish (7" x 11" works well). Combine melted butter and crumbs. Sprinkle on top. Bake 25 minutes at 375°.

In a sauté pan heat 1 tsp. of coconut oil, add the rainbow chard, sea salt or tamari, and leave for about one minute until wilted. Serve hot over the turnip puff.

Sunshine Raw Vegetarian Nori Rolls

Instead of rice, this recipe uses sunflower seeds that are much richer in protein, fiber, and good fat making this meal balanced and protein dense unlike most veggie nori rolls. They are easy to make once you get the hang of it, and you can experiment with the inside ingredients as you get comfortable with the process.

½ cups hulled sunflower seeds

½ mango sliced into long strips

2 green onions, green parts only, chopped and divided

2 tbsp. lime juice

2 tbsp. tamari

1 clove garlic

3 small collard green leaves

3 sheets nori

1 cucumber, peeled, seeded, and cut into strips

1 avocado, halved and thinly sliced

Soak the sunflower seeds in cold filtered water for a couple of hours. Place the soaked seeds into the food processor with the tamari, garlic, lime juice, and half the green onions. Blend into a smooth paste. Place the nori sheets flat on a cutting board, line with one leaf of collard greens. Spread about 2 tablespoons of sunflower paste onto collards (a spatula works well). Then down one side stack the cucumber, avocado, mango and remaining green onion so it makes a line from top to bottom. Roll the strips up until tight as you can and dab some water along the edge to seal. Cut into 1 inch pieces and serve. Dip in tamari if you like and enjoy.

Heirloom Gazpacho, Spanish Quinoa and Avocado Salad

This is a delicious recipe especially in season when you can get some plump juicy garden tomatoes. The quinoa substitution for the rice is a great way to up the protein, and the whole thing finished off with a dollop of avocado salad is just perfect.

Gazpacho:

3 pounds ripe heirloom tomatoes
1 clove garlic
2 tsp. salt
4 tbp. olive oil
2 tbsp. good quality wine vinegar
½ green pepper (Italian, long thin)
2 cucumbers
½ small onion
1 cup water

Optional garnish to serve on top of soup:

½ small onion chopped
½ green pepper chopped
½ cucumber chopped
1 small tomato chopped

Place heirloom tomatoes in the blender until they are pureed. Strain to take away the skin and seeds. Put the remainder of the ingredients into the blender with the tomato puree, garlic, salt, cucumber, onion and pepper. Process until pureed, with the motor running, add the oil in a slow stream, and then add the vinegar.

The mixture will thicken and change color as the oil emulsifies. Stir in the water. Chill until serving time. If the soup is too thick, stir in more tomato juice or water. Garnish with any of the optional suggestions.

Spanish Quinoa:

1 cup cooked quinoa
½ cup small onion, chopped
½ cup medium green
   pepper, chopped
1 tbsp. butter

4 oz. tomato sauce or diced
   tomatoes
2 mild green chilies
   (optional)
¼ tsp. sea salt

Simmer the onion, pepper, green chili, and sea salt together in butter in a hot skillet until cooked and soft. Toss into cooked quinoa and stir in tomato sauce.

Avocado Salad:

1 avocado
½ cup cucumber, chopped
¼ cup fresh red onion,
   chopped (optional)

¼ cup cilantro, chopped
juice from half a lime
sea salt to taste

Coarsely chop the cucumber, and avocado. Finely chop the onion and cilantro. Mix gently into a bowl to keep the avocado from mashing. Sprinkle with lime juice and sea salt

Roasted Fig and Goat Cheese Salad

This is a delicious salad for a light meal. It has both chevre and sprouted pumpkin seeds for protein. Sprouted seeds are more nutrient dense than unsprouted seeds, so if you can find them it is worth it, or you can sprout your own.

⅓ cup apple cider vinegar
1 tbsp. molasses
2 tsp. extra virgin olive oil
2 tbsp. sea salt
4 large fresh figs, cut in half
1–2 handfuls of organic
    greens

2 oz. chevre (soft goat
    cheese)
Course ground black pepper
¼ cup sprouted pumpkin
    seeds

Combine first 4 ingredients in a medium bowl, stirring with a whisk. Add figs and toss to coat. Remove figs with a slotted spoon, reserving vinegar mixture.

Place figs in a cast-iron or ovenproof skillet. Bake at 425° for 8 to 10 minutes. Remove figs from pan and place on a plate. Immediately add reserved vinegar mixture to the hot pan, scraping pan to loosen browned bits. Pour into a small bowl. Let figs and vinaigrette cool to room temperature.

Place salad greens on a platter. Arrange figs over greens and sprinkle with chevre and pepper. Gently mix in sprouted pumpkin seeds. Drizzle with cooled vinaigrette.

Tortilla Espanola and Arugula Salad

Tortilla Espanola or Spanish omelet is the most commonly served dish in Spain. This single-serving recipe can be increased proportionally to accommodate a large party or enough for leftovers.

Tortilla:

1–2 eggs, beaten
Salt to taste
1–2 tbsp. olive oil
1 small red potatoes (lower glycemic), peeled and thinly sliced

1 onion, peeled and finely chopped
green olives, chopped for garnish

Heat olive oil in a frying pan. If you are making one serving, a very small pan is best. Add the potato and fry for a couple of minutes until it starts to turn golden. Add the onion and mix together in the frying pan. Meanwhile, crack the egg(s) into a bowl and whisk with a bit of salt. When the potato and onion are golden brown add the egg(s). Make sure the potato and onions are fully covered by the eggs. Fry this gently on low heat for 3-4 minutes. While it is cooking, free the sides and the bottom with a spatula, so it is easier to remove. Once it is lightly browned on the bottom, place a plate upside down over the frying pan. With one hand on the frying pan handle and the other on top of the plate to hold it steady, quickly turn the frying pan over and the omelet will fall onto the plate. If you want to fry the other side, place the frying pan back on the range and put just enough oil to cover the bottom and sides of the pan. Let the pan warm for 30 seconds or so. Then slide the omelet back into the frying pan. Use the spatula to shape the sides of the omelet. Let the omelet cook for 3-4 minutes. Turn the heat off and let the tortilla sit in the pan for 2 minutes. Turn the pan over and place the tortilla on a serving plate. Let it settle for about 5 to 7 minutes before serving. Garnish with green olives, which is a Spanish tradition. It is also delicious with tomato sauce.

Salad:

2 cups arugula, washed and chopped
¼ cup tomato, chopped

1 tbsp. flax oil
squeeze from ½ a lemon
sea salt to taste

Mix together the arugula and the fresh tomatoes. Drizzle with flax oil, lemon and salt to taste. Serve alongside the tortilla.

ARE YOU READY? _____

**Contact Us to Talk With One of Our
Nutritional Cleansing Coaches for Free**

We make sure you don't do this without the support of a nutritional cleansing coach at no cost.

Your free coach will help you take each step you need to ensure a healthier you and assist you in living healthier, longer.

We await your call:

800-931-7810

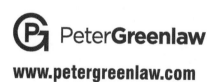

www.petergreenlaw.com

Made in the USA
Charleston, SC
12 November 2012